Neighborhoods

Impact on Child Health and Development

nova
Medicine & Health
New York

Public Health: Practices, Methods and Policies Series

Joav Merrick - Series Editor

Medical Director, Health Services, Division for Intellectual and Developmental Disabilities, Ministry of Social Affairs and Social Services, Jerusalem, Israel

Environmental Health: Social and Environmental Determinants of Health
I. Leslie Rubin, MD and
Joav Merrick, MD, MMedSci, DMSc
(Editors)
ISBN: 979-8-89530-748-9
eBook ISBN: 979-8-89530-780-9

COVID-19: Service-Learning in a Chinese Context
Betty Mok, DSW,
Daniel T.L. Shek, PhD, FHKPS, BBS, SBS, JP, and
Joav Merrick, MD, MMedSci, DMSc
(Editors)
ISBN: 979-8-89530-743-4
eBook ISBN: 979-8-89530-787-8

Public Health: Audiology Research in Malaysia
Mohd N. Zakaria, PhD and
Joav Merrick, MD, MMedSci, DMSc
(Editors)
ISBN: 979-8-89530-577-5
eBook ISBN: 979-8-89530-663-5

Hong Kong and China: Promotion of Holistic Development in Young People Under the Service Economy
Daniel T.L. Shek, PhD, FHKPS, BBS, SBS, JP, Xiaoqin Zhu, PhD,
Diya Dou, PhD, Xiang Li, PhD and
Joav Merrick, MD, MMedSci, DMSc
(Editors)
ISBN: 979-8-89530-747-2
eBook ISBN: 979-8-89530-794-6

Public Health: Understanding the Impact of Environmental Pollutants
Emmanuel Obeng-Gyasi, PhD, MPH
and Joav Merrick, MD, MMedSci, DMSc (Editors)
ISBN: 979-8-89530-579-9
eBook ISBN: 979-8-89530-636-9

More information about this series can be found at
https://novapublishers.com/product-category/series/public-health-practices-methods-and-policies/

I Leslie Rubin
and Joav Merrick
Editors

Neighborhoods

Impact on Child Health and Development

nova
Medicine & Health
New York

DOI: https://doi.org/10.52305/QAGX8342

Library of Congress Cataloging-in-Publication Data
Library of Congress Control Number: 2025947429
ISBN: 979-8-89530-834-9 (Hardcover)
ISBN: 979-8-89530-909-4 (eBook)

Published by Nova Science Publishers, Inc. † New York

Contents

Introduction

Chapter 1

Break the Cycle of children's environmental health disparities program and student projects: The social, psychological, emotional, educational and environmental determinants of health

I Leslie Rubin, MD[1-5],
Abby Mutic, APRN, PhD[3,6]
Victoria Green, JD, MD[3,7]
Melissa Gittinger, DO[3,8]
Jinbing Bai, PhD, RN[3,6]
Nathan Mutic[3,6]
Wayne Garfinkel, BSCE[3,8]
Henry Falk, MD, MPH[3,4]
Benjamin A Gitterman, MD[9,10]
Martha Berge[11]
Stacie Schmidt[12,13]
and Joav Merrick, MD, MMedSci, DMSc[14-17]

[1]Department of Pediatrics, Morehouse School of Medicine, Atlanta, Georgia, United States of America
[2]Department of Pediatrics, Emory University School of Medicine, Atlanta, Georgia, United States of America
[3]Southeast Pediatric Environmental Health Specialty Unit, Emory University, Atlanta, Georgia, United States of America
[4]Break the Cycle of Health Disparities Inc, Atlanta, Georgia, United States of America

In: Neighborhoods: Impact on Child Health and Development
Editors: I Leslie Rubin and Joav Merrick
ISBN: 979-8-89530-834-9

[5]The Rubin Center for Autism and Developmental Pediatrics, Atlanta, Georgia, United States of America
[6]Nell Hodgson Woodruff School of Nursing, Emory University, Atlanta, Georgia, United States of America
[7]Department of Gynecology and Obstetrics, Emory University School of Medicine, Atlanta, Georgia, United States of America
[8]Retired EPA Region 4 Children's Environmental Health Coordinator, Atlanta, Georgia, United States of America
[9]Departments of Pediatrics and Public Health, George Washington University Schools of Medicine and Public Health and Health Services, Washington, D.C., United States of America
[10]General and Community Pediatrics, Children's National Medical Center, Washington DC, United States of America
[11]Climate Equity Collaborative
[12]Department of Medicine, Emory University School of Medicine, Atlanta, Georgia, United States of America
[13]Grady Health Systems
[14]National Institute of Child Health and Human Development, Jerusalem, Israel
[15]Division of Pediatrics, Hadassah Hebrew University Medical Center, Mt Scopus Campus, Jerusalem, Israel
[16]Kentucky Children's Hospital, University of Kentucky College of Medicine, Lexington, Kentucky, United States of America
[17]Center for Human Development, School of Public Health, Georgia State University, Atlanta, Georgia, United States of America

The impact of poverty on children's physical and mental health, and on their education has profound long term and intergenerational consequences in limited employment options and limited income, with limited residential options to older houses in more crowded neighborhoods. In these settings, there is an increased risk of exposure to environmental toxins, like lead and air pollution, with adverse physical and mental health outcomes, particularly for children, which, along with limited access to quality healthcare, further compromises children's health and function, thus limiting future opportunities for success and perpetuating the plight of poverty. This intergenerational pattern can be represented as a *Cycle of Health Disparities,* which provides a conceptual framework for developing intervention strategies. *Break the Cycle of Children's Environmental Health Disparities* is an annual, collaborative interdisciplinary research and training program for university students, who recognize the impact of adverse social, economic, and environmental factors on children's health, growth, learning, development and engage in creative projects to *Break the Cycle* and reduce children's health disparities and, in the process, they gain insight and skills to become future leaders in our society. The projects from the students who participated in our 18th Annual *Break the Cycle* program are featured in this book.

Abbreviations

PEHSU – Pediatric Environmental Health Specialty Unit
SDOH – Social Determinants of Health

Introduction

Measures of societal health can be seen in access to clean safe drinking water, nutritious food, quality education, quality healthcare, opportunities for gainful employment, functional participation in society, social and cultural community engagement, and access to resources for recreation. When all these needs are met, the reports on quality of life and feelings of wellbeing are positive, there is a sense of purpose and value, resulting in achievement and productivity, that then enhances and perpetuates the positivity.

The health and wellbeing of a society can be measured in per capita income, productivity and in life expectancy, which are all related and interactive. It is notable and promising that life expectancy has increased globally from about 40-50 years in the early 1950's to over 70 years in the 2020's (1). The factors that have contributed to the increase in life expectancy worldwide are related to improved sanitation and access to clean water, access to healthy food and improved nutrition, effective disease prevention programs, quality healthcare, and advancements in medical technology, along with reduced poverty, increased education levels, government policies reducing exposure to potentially harmful environmental factors, and public health policies promoting healthy lifestyles.

Global disparities in life expectancy and child mortality

While this increase in life expectancy is reported across all counties, it is by no means equitable. Obviously, the countries with greater per capita income, and more stable societies and governments will have a longer life expectancy than countries with lower per capita income and less stable societies. Countries with the highest life expectancy (in the 85-90-year range) are in Monaco,

Singapore, Macau and Japan, while the countries with the lowest life expectancy (in the 55-60-year range) are in Afghanistan and counties in sub-Saharan Africa, Central African Republic, Somalia, Mozambique and Sierra Leone (2). Thus, although progress has been made in global life expectancy there are major disparities related to income, resources, social infrastructure and political stability.

While the general health of a population can be measured in life expectancy, the health and well-being of children is measured in infant and child mortality. Parallel to the improvement in life expectancy for the general population over the past decades as a result of improved access to clean water and good nutrition, as well as in public health and prevention of diseases, improved quality of healthcare and advances in medical technology, there has been a reduction in infant and child mortality. Globally, the under-five child mortality rate declined from 93 deaths per 1,000 live births in 1990 to 37 deaths per 1,000 live births in 2022. Like the global distribution statistics on life expectancy by country, the measure of child health in child under-five mortality rate by country is at a dramatically low around 1-2 per 1,000 live births in Japan and Scandinavian countries, while it is disturbingly high at 90-100 per 1,000 live births in Afghanistan and countries in Sub-Sharan Africa (3).

Disparities in child mortality in the United States

While the lowest global under-five child mortality rate is in the 1-2 per 1,000 live birth rage, the United States (US) rate is at 5-6 per 1,000 live births, which ranks in the mid 50's by country and in a range similar to countries like Bulgaria, Bosnia, Chile and Saudi Arabia (4). The question may be asked, why is the child mortality in the US so high, when it is a wealthy country with a high per capita income and a stable society with good infrastructure? The reason is that, although the child mortality rate for children from affluent families in the US is relatively low, the mortality rate for children from poor families is relatively high, in fact, more than double that of their more affluent counterparts.

The CDC reports on infant mortality by state, which corresponds in part to the state per capita income (5, 6). Out of all 50 states, New York had the highest per-capita real gross domestic product (GDP) in 2023, at $90,730, followed by Massachusetts at $87.860 and Washington at $87,027 and California at $82,975. The states with the lowest per-capita real GDP were

Alabama at $47,393, Arkansas at $45,892, West Virginia at $45,272, and the lowest in Mississippi at $39,102, and (7) (see figure 1). It should also be noted that the poorest states have the highest percentage of Black people, with in Mississippi having 38% Black people, Louisiana has 34%, Georgia 32%, Maryland 32%, Alabama 27%, and South Carolina 26% (8). Black children are three times more likely to be poor (9) and have a child mortality more than double that of white children at around 10 per 1,000 live births and a mortality rate from asthma that is almost 8 times that of White youth (10).

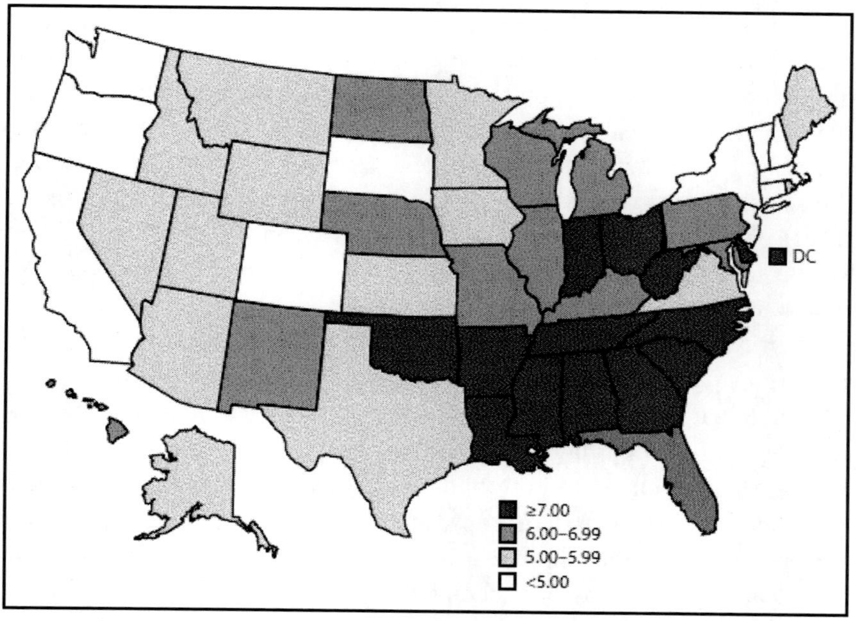

Figure 1. Infant mortality rate in the United States by state (CDC).

Income disparities and child health in the United States

It should be noted that relative poverty or affluence is directly linked to parental education which clearly determines the type of employment and corresponding income and is linked child mortality (11). The association of family income with child health and mortality rate can be understood in the context of what a substantial income can bring to a family and what would be lacking or absent from a family with limited income.

For families with predictable source of income, living in a comfortable home in a safe neighborhood, with enough food on the table for them and for their children, and having access to good neighborhood schools, and health insurance that will cover medical expenses and measures of social capital, they can feel secure about their situation and enjoy good health for themselves and for their children. In contrast, families who are poor are more likely to face the stresses of day-to-day life in a survival mode. They may have to worry about a dependable source of income, their ability to put food on the table, to have a secure and safe place to live, in a relatively safe neighborhood, the necessary resources to deal with unexpected illnesses that would require medical attention and take time away from work, risking potentially reduced income, caring for the health and wellbeing of their children, making sure their children have enough food to eat, clean clothes to wear, and that they are safe, and they have a good education that will help them get good jobs and have a measure of financial security when they become adults. These insecurities are stressful and can stimulate the hormones of stress that can adversely affect their physical and emotional wellbeing and further complicate and compound their stresses and existing adversities (12).

Their children, in turn, grow up experiencing the stresses of their parents, and their own adverse experiences that influence their physical and emotional health and their education (13). They may experience housing insecurity and may have to move more often, they may experience eviction and homelessness, they may suffer from food insecurity, they may be neglected or abused and suffer the long-term consequences. They may live in older houses with lead paint with the risk of lead poisoning that causes brain damage and affects learning and behavior, reducing the likelihood of doing well at school (14). They may live in houses where the heating and air-conditioning systems are not functioning optimally and increase the risk of asthma, and they may live in neighborhoods where there is much traffic and air pollution further increasing the likelihood of asthma (15). They may live in neighborhoods that are crowded with limited green space for recreations, or there are drugs and crime on the streets making it risky to go outdoors and may choose to stay home and watch TV or play video games (16). Their neighborhoods are more likely to be ‘food deserts’ with limited availability of fresh produce and good food choices, so they must rely on the fast-food franchises with high sugar, high salt, high calorie foods that are limited in essential nutrients, or food from convenience stores that have high levels of preservatives and artificial ingredients. As a result, they are more likely to become obese (17) with the potential metabolic consequences of diabetes, as well as cardiovascular complications of hypertension, limiting and their level of physical activity and becoming more sedentary, which further contributes to their obesity, and the associated emotional and mental health consequences with poor self-esteem and increased potential for depression (18).

The schools they attend are more likely to be old and have poorly functioning heating and air conditioning systems creating a less than comfortable learning environment. Furthermore, in poor neighborhoods the teachers are paid less and may be less enthusiastic about teaching so the students are not stimulated as much to learn, which can impact the likelihood of graduating and increasing the dropout rate, with those children less likely to secure good paying jobs and more likely to be unemployed thus perpetuating their state of poverty (19). For those students who do go on to graduate, because they may not have had a quality education, they may not be able to get as well-paying jobs as their counterparts who have gone to good schools and are better prepared and qualified to secure compete for higher paying jobs (20).

Furthermore, many children who come from this stressful background are more likely to suffer from learning disabilities, ADHD and mental health disorders such as depression (21), and they have limited access to quality healthcare. They live in neighborhoods where there may be drugs and crime, where they are more likely to engage in drug use and to secure enough money to buy the drugs, they may resort to selling drugs or commit crime that may result in arrests and incarceration (22). Also, because of the higher prevalence of crime in the poorer neighborhoods, there is more likely to be violence and access to firearms, resulting in increasing rates of homicides and suicides. Interestingly, considering that poverty is greater among Black children compared to White children which translates into these residential realities, the homicide rate in Black youth between 2016-2020 was 10 times that of White youth, and the firearm mortality rate for Black youth was four times that of White youth (10).

Poor young women are more likely to become pregnant as teenagers, especially if they had also experienced neglect or abuse (23). Furthermore, because many may be using tobacco, alcohol or other drugs, not only is the fetus is likely more likely to be born premature, they are also more likely to be adversely affected by toxic effects of the drugs on brain development with significant neurodevelopmental consequences, such as ADHD, learning disabilities, and behavior problems (24). These children will already have a disadvantage even before they enter the family, community and neighborhood characterized by poverty and its associated litany of adverse impacts and their respective consequences.

Cycle of health disparities

As can be seen in the above descriptions, the impact of poverty on children's physical and mental health, and on education and opportunity, results in limited employment options, limited income, with limited residential options, to older houses and more crowded neighborhoods with increased risk of exposure to environmental pollutants, like lead and air pollution that have adverse health outcomes, along with limited access to quality healthcare that further compromises health and function, particularly of their children. This intergenerational pattern can be conceptualized in a Cycle of Health Disparities (see figure 2). Although the perpetuating cycle may seem daunting if not insurmountable, much progress has been made at many levels in understanding the relationships between poverty and health, social determinants of health, environmental factors that adversely affect health, impact of racial discrimination on health, the importance of education, awareness of the critical necessity of health care for all, impacts of government policies, proliferation of non-governmental organizations, principles of collaboration between organizations and agencies, the value of philanthropies and, significantly, that of human resilience.

Into this mix of strategies to improve the health of vulnerable children and help them reach their full potential as functioning contributing members of society, we have established a program called *Break the Cycle of Children's Environmental Health Disparities*.

Break the cycle program

Break the Cycle of Children's Environmental Health Disparities is an annual, collaborative interdisciplinary research and training program for university students who recognize the impact of adverse social, economic, and environmental factors on children's health, growth, learning, development and future as active contributing citizens in society. Each participating student engages in a creative project that focuses on improving the health, growth and development of children who live in communities where stresses related to circumstances of social and economic disadvantage are compounded by exposure to toxic chemical hazards. What makes this program unique is that each student must view his or her project in the ecological framework of the Cycle of Health Disparities. This adds dimension and perspective to the project and provides the student with a world view that is multifaceted and more comprehensive (see figure 2).

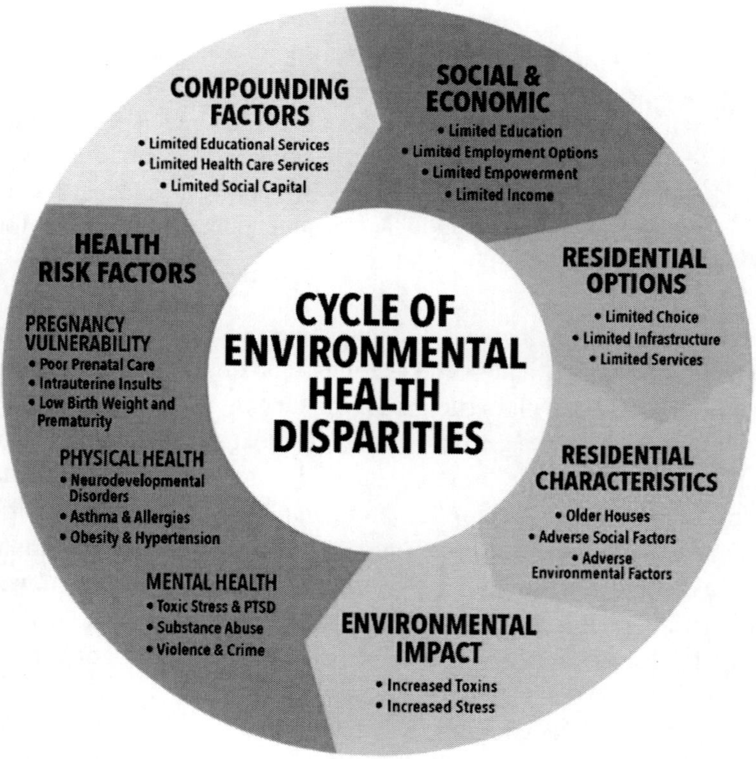

Figure 2. Cycle of environmental health disparities (25).

During the process, the students work on their projects with their university faculty mentors and report their progress on a monthly basis in group sessions to the *Break the Cycle* faculty. As part of the review sessions, they are presented with a curriculum of in-depth relevant topics to illustrate and support the concepts embedded in the cycle of health disparities, such as social determinants of health, environmental justice, community engagement, health literacy, and health communication. At the completion of their projects, the students are expected present their findings at a national conference and then write up their projects for publication in an international journal.

The goal of working with the students is twofold:

- The one goal is practical and *quantitative*: to support the students in the completion of their projects, to help them to prepare their completed work for presentation at the annual conference, and assist them in writing a manuscript of their work for publication.
- The other goal is *qualitative*: to enable them to appreciate the ecological context of children's environmental health that encompasses the historical, political, economic, social and environmental determinants of health, and how they can make a significant difference in improving children's health, and empower them to become future leaders in promoting health equity for all children and improving societal health in the present and for the future.

It is also anticipated that participating students will inspire their peers in academic, professional, and social settings, and that the interdisciplinary nature of the program with participation of students from other universities, disciplines and perspectives, offers a greater context and understanding of the complexities of children's health disparities and how they can play a productive and transformative role. Through cultivating the natural curiosity and talents of the students and providing them with the necessary information, insights and strategies along with a sense of purpose and mission, towards a goal of providing vulnerable children with greater opportunities to reach their full potential, the students will become productive and contributing members and future leaders in our society.

The variety of student projects represented in this volume offers a sampling of the diversity of perspectives on the elements inherent in children's environmental health disparities and how each can make a positive difference, thereby, enhancing our collective knowledge of children's environmental health and environmental health disparities. Through this process, each student gains knowledge and experience in the research process, and, with exposure to different perspectives from the other student projects, equips them to become advocates for improving the health and wellbeing of vulnerable children.

Break the cycle student projects

Since its inception in 2004, *Break the Cycle* has held 17 annual programs and worked with over 180 students representing 50 different university departments in 21 states in the United States, as well as students from countries in Latin America, Europe, and Africa. To date, manuscripts of student projects have been published in 16 monographs in international journals and 16 books in a public health series (25).

Below are the abstracts of the student projects from our 18th Annual Break the Cycle program. The diversity of topics in this small sample gives an idea of the advantage of examining the different aspects of the lives of vulnerable children and inspires us all to continue to be creative in breaking the cycle of children's environmental disparities.

Examining the impact of adverse childhood experiences on educational outcomes of students with an emotional behavior disorder

Nicole Houston, BS, MEd and Miles Anthony Irving, PhD
Department of Learning Sciences, College of Education and Human Development, Georgia State University, Atlanta, Georgia, United States of America

Abstract: The impact of multiple adverse childhood experiences (ACEs) on a child's health and development is well known. In the field of education, ACEs have been studied to help understand students with problematic internalizing and externalizing behaviors. To date, research has not explored the association and impact of ACEs among students who qualify to receive additional school supports through individualized education plan (IEP) in the category of emotional behavior disorder (EBD). Among all disability subgroups identified in the school setting, students with EBD experience the most negative behavioral, educational and long-term outcomes while in school and after graduation. Due to systemically inequitable policies impacting minority communities, Black children are disproportionately identified as having EBD, as well as disproportionately experiencing multiple ACEs. We undertook a literature review to summarize prior research assessing behavioral, educational, and long-term outcomes of students with ACEs and students with EBD separately and explore the relationship between experiences and outcomes of children experiencing multiple ACEs and students with EBD. Our findings reveal many overlapping outcomes in the areas of education and adult health outcomes. Future research to study the relationships between ACEs and EBD is recommended for communities and schools to provide adequate resources to students who have significant behavioral challenges, especially Black students who are disproportionately affected by ACEs and disproportionately represented by EBD. Such research and resource development could serve to help break the cycle of racial disparities and inequities that impact educational performance and postsecondary outcomes, to provide the students with a promising future.

Neighborhood child opportunity, air pollution and telomere length among children

Austin Le, MS[1], Stephanie Holm, MD, PhD, MPH[2], Morgan Ye, MPH[3], Nicole R Bush, PhD[4,5], Danielle Hessler, PhD[6], Kadiatou Koita, MD, MS[7], Monica Bucci, MD[7], Dayna Long, MD[5,8], Neeta Thakur, MD, MPH[3] and Rosemarie de la Rosa, PhD, MPH[1,3]

[1]Environmental Health Sciences Division, School of Public Health, University of California, Berkeley, [2]Western States Pediatric Environmental Health Specialty Unit, San Francisco, [3]Division of Pulmonary and Critical Care Medicine, Department of Medicine, University of California, San Francisco, [4]Department of Psychiatry and Behavioral Science, University of California, San Francisco, [5]Department of Pediatrics, University of California, San Francisco, [6]Department of Family and Community Medicine, University of California, San Francisco, [7]Center for Youth Wellness, San Francisco and [8]UCSF Benioff Children's Hospital Oakland, San Francisco, California, United States of America

Abstract: Neighborhood resources are associated with positive health outcomes among children. Telomere length (TL) serves as a marker of stress-related, biological aging and inversely associated with adverse environmental factors. Objective: Examine the association between neighborhood child opportunity and residential ambient air pollution with TL among children and assess whether this association is modified by neighborhood child opportunity. Study group: Children (1-11 years of age) from the Pediatric Adverse Childhood Experiences (ACEs) and Resiliency Study cohort. Methods: Neighborhood Child Opportunity Index (COI) and ambient particulate matter

($PM_{2.5}$) concentrations were matched to residential locations for the twelve months prior to biospecimen collection. Relative buccal TL was measured using quantitative polymerase chain reaction. Multivariable linear regression models were used to examine for associations between neighborhood COI (continuous and categorical) and TL, adjusting for sociodemographics. Results: The study sample consisted of 299 children (45.8% girls, mean age of 6.0 years [standard deviation: 3.4]) with median COI of 28.0 [IQR: 41.5], median 12-month prior $PM_{2.5}$ concentrations of 11.8 μg/m^3 [IQR: 2.5], and median TL of 0.1 [IQR: 0.03]. Continuous and categorical COI and COI domains were not associated with TL. Average 12-month prior residential $PM_{2.5}$ was associated with shorter TL (ß = -0.02, 95% CI: -0.04, -0.01). The interaction between COI and $PM_{2.5}$ exposure on TL was nonsignificant ($p = 0.82$). Conclusions: Neighborhood resources were not found to have an impact on physiologic aging among young children. Future longitudinal studies are warranted to explore the long-term impact of neighborhood environments on health outcomes as children advance into adolescence and adulthood.

Evaluating the effectiveness of pandemic-era anti-eviction policies on children's health

Anna McPeak and John Marshall, JD
College of Law, Georgia State University, Atlanta, Georgia, United States of America

Abstract: Evictions result in a myriad of health and mental problems for adults and children alike. The impacts of eviction on children include displacement, health risks, and behavioral problems. These outcomes have not been well documented, and data is thus unavailable to policymakers when making laws. In 2021, a handful of states implemented statutory changes to alleviate the pressure tenants often feel upon receiving notice of an eviction. This paper seeks to evaluate 1) the effectiveness of statutory changes on children's health, 2) rates of tenant confidence in ability to pay rent in states that imposed these new laws and 3) whether these laws had any impact on poverty rates. Additionally, this study postulates how these laws can have impact, and findings will guide future studies of eviction impacts on children's health.

The relationship between race and access to public water and sewer service in Halifax County, North Carolina

Banks Grubbs, BSPH and Jacqueline MacDonald Gibson, PhD
Department of Civil, Construction, and Environmental Engineering, North Carolina State University, Raleigh, North Carolina, United States of America

Abstract: Numerous studies have shown that Black communities on the fringes of Southern towns and cities in the United States have been systematically denied access to critical infrastructure such as public water and sewer services. This research investigates the relationship between race and access to these services within the six extraterritorial jurisdictions (ETJs) of Halifax County, North Carolina. Utilizing multivariate logistic regressions, the relationship between the proportion of Black people living in a census block and the odds of a residence in that block having public water or sewer access was estimated. Significant negative relationships were identified between the proportion of Black people per census block and odds of access to public water in the ETJs of Roanoke Rapids (OR = 0.24, $p = 0.0237$) and Littleton (OR = 0.025, $p = 0.0162$), and the odds of access to sewer service in the ETJs of Roanoke Rapids (OR = 0.04, $p<0.001$), Littleton (OR = 0.027, $p = 0.0162$), and Scotland Neck (OR = 0.259, $p = 0.032$). These results suggest that predominantly Black communities in these ETJs are less likely to have access to public water and sewer services. People who do not have access to these services are more likely to rely on private wells and septic systems, which are associated with increased exposure to contaminants like lead and disease-causing microorganisms. Therefore, these excluded communities are potentially more likely to be exposed to harmful environmental contaminants and to experience related negative health outcomes, contributing to a cycle of environmental health disparities.

School garden model strategies to combat food insecurity in Lumpkin County, Georgia

Jami Nakan, BS[1,2], Julie Knight-Brown, MS[1] and David Patterson, PhD[2]
[1]*Lumpkin County School District, Lumpkin County, Georgia and* [2]*Department of Biology, The University of North Georgia, Dahlonega, Georgia, United States of America*

Abstract: Food insecurity, as defined by the United States Department of Agriculture, is "a household-level economic and social condition of limited or uncertain access to adequate food." According to the Georgia Department of Education, nearly half of the kindergarten through twelfth-grade students in the Lumpkin County School System in Northeast Georgia are impacted by food insecurity. To address this issue, classes from a local elementary school in Lumpkin County participated in a small-scale garden project designed to provide students with agricultural education and fresh produce from an on-site garden. Classroom evaluations demonstrate that the project was effective in teaching fifth-grade students basic STEM topics centered on garden activities, including botany, physiology, and agricultural practices, while also providing a source of fresh produce. This model offers a simple and effective strategy to address childhood food insecurity and sustainable agricultural education in rural districts in Georgia.

Presence of stressors surrounding local elementary schools in redlined and non-redlined communities in Albany, New York, November–December 2022

Kaylee Stewart and Stacy M Pettigrew, BA, MS, PhD
Albany College of Pharmacy and Health Sciences, Albany, New York, United States of America

Abstract: Lending patterns based on the 1933 Home Owners' Loan Corporation map characterizations resulted in long lasting and persistent economic and racial disparities. Many neighborhoods deemed 'hazardous' at the time remain low-income today. Poverty can increase children's stress levels, which can result in adverse health effects from childhood into adulthood.

Objective: To determine differences in the presence of stressors surrounding redlined and non-redlined schools in Albany, New York. Methods: Data collection consisted of two components: (i) an observational study that evaluated the non-permanent stressors that the students were exposed to and (ii) a mapping identification to locate and evaluate stressors that students were seeing on a regular basis. The Kruskal Wallis one-way analysis of variance was used to test differences between individual schools and by redlining map status. Results: Preliminary data were collected during cold months. No significant difference was observed ($p = 0.178$) between the stressors around schools in redlined versus non-redlined neighborhoods. However, one of the two schools located in a redlined neighborhood did have a significantly greater ($p = 0.0295$) number of stressors compared to the other schools. Conclusion: Statistically significant differences in stressors by redlined status were not observed in this limited analysis. However, a difference in the presence of stressors [found] between the two redlined schools could be due to differences in the built environment surrounding each school, such as street traffic and green space. Data collection will be repeated in May and September to increase sample size and capture the stressors during warmer months.

Increased maternal education weakens the link between maternal health during pregnancy and adverse child health outcomes later in life

Margaret Pinder, BSPH[1], Kyle R Roell, PhD[1,2], T Michael O'Shea, MD, MPH[3] and Rebecca C Fry, MS, PhD[1,2,4]
[1]Department of Environmental Health Sciences and [2]The Institute for Environmental Health Solutions, Gillings School of Global Public Health, University of North Carolina at Chapel Hill, Chapel Hill, North Carolina, [3]Department of Pediatrics, Division of Neonatal-Perinatal Medicine, University of North Carolina, Chapel Hill, North Carolina and [4]Curriculum in Toxicology and Environmental Medicine, School of Medicine, University of North Carolina, Chapel Hill, North Carolina, United States of America

Abstract: Research from the extremely low gestational age newborn (ELGAN) study of children born earlier than 28 weeks' gestation indicates that maternal health conditions during pregnancy are associated with worse health in the offspring. Using extant data from the ELGAN Study we evaluated whether increased years of maternal education between birth and age 15 years moderated the relationship between maternal health conditions and child health at age 15 years. At the time of birth, data were collected about maternal health conditions, including pre-pregnancy diabetes, obesity, hypertension, and asthma. When the ELGAN participants were two, ten, and fifteen years old, data were collected about the number of years of formal education completed by the mother. Based on data about child health outcomes at 15 years of age, a positive child health index (PCHI) was developed, with higher PCHI indicating more positive health. Among study participants (n = 694), 21% were born at 23-24 weeks of gestation, 46% at 25-26 weeks, and 33% at 27 weeks. years of age). Fifty-one percent of participants were male. Sixty-three percent of mothers had reached at least some college education at the time of the ELGAN participant's birth, and 42% had additional years of formal education during their child's first 15 years of life. Three maternal health conditions at birth (asthma, obesity, and diabetes) were associated with worse child health at age 15; maternal hypertension was not associated with child health at age 15. In stratified analysis, associations between maternal asthma, obesity, and diabetes and worse child health were weaker among study participants whose mothers completed additional formal education between the child's birth and the child's study visit at 15 years.

Conclusion

The consequences of poverty on the health and well-being of children are evident in the dramatic disparities in health and in access to quality healthcare. Income-related disparities are compounded and multiplied by the impact of discriminatory practices at many levels. The human costs in loss of earning potential and the added economic costs to society in supporting such large populations of poor children in poor physical, social, and emotional health, take its toll on the whole of society. It is, therefore, incumbent upon us to recognize the resultant costs in loss in human potential for the individual and for society, and to continue to develop creative strategies to reduce the disparities and promote health equity for all children. In this spirit, we offer our *Break the Cycle* program as a model for university students to develop creative and productive projects to reduce children's health disparities and, in the process, cultivate their potential to become future leaders to make positive changes to our society.

As a core principle, *Break the Cycle* promotes awareness of the social, economic, and environmental determinants of health and encourages university students to develop creative and innovative strategies to reduce and eliminate children's health disparities in our society for the good of all. Students who participate in our annual *Break the Cycle* programs, benefit from the process of creatively conceptualizing and developing a project, translating it into action, performing the research, presenting the results of their projects at a national conference, and writing manuscripts for publication in this journal. Each student project highlights different ways to *Break the Cycle of*

Children's Environmental Health Disparities through different components of the *Break the Cycle* diagram (see figure 2).

In this process, the students gain valuable knowledge and skills towards becoming the next generation of leaders, and, building on their knowledge and experience, to further the goals of reducing children's environmental health disparities and promoting health equity for all children. This research and training model is a relatively inexpensive and cost-effective way of inspiring bright young students to focus their potential on changing the world for the better by stimulating their creativity, encouraging and enhancing their research and communication skills, and by embodying the principles of justice, equity, and collaboration. In the process, we all gain additional knowledge, understanding and perspective to become more inclusive and open to positive innovations and progress.

Acknowledgements

Thanks to the additional editors of some of the papers who have given of their time and expertise, much appreciated especially our trusted friend and star guest editor, David Ervin, at Makom in Baltimore, Samantha Lange at the University of Johannesburg, South Africa, Laura Anderko, at the Villanova University and Mid-Atlantic PEHSU, and Robert Geller at the Department of Pediatrics at Emory University. This publication was supported by the cooperative agreement award number 5 NU61TS000237-05 from the Agency for Toxic Substances and Disease Registry (ATSDR). Its contents are the responsibility of the authors and do not necessarily represent the official views of the Agency for Toxic Substances and Disease Registry (ATSDR). The US Environmental Protection Agency (EPA) supports the PEHSU by providing partial funding to ATSDR under Inter-Agency Agreement number DW-75-95877701. Neither EPA nor ATSDR endorse the purchase of any commercial products or services mentioned in PEHSU publications.

References

[1] United Nations Population Division. Mortality. URL: https://www.un.org/development/desa/pd/content/mortality-0.

[2] The World Factbook. Life expectancy at birth. URL: https://www.cia.gov/the-world-factbook/field/life-expectancy-at-birth/country-comparison/.

[3] World Health Organization. Under 5 mortality rate per 1,000 live births. URL: https://www.who.int/data/gho/data/indicators/indicator-details/GHO/under-five-mortality-rate-(probability-of-dying-by-age-5-per-1000-live-births).

[4] UNICEF for Every Child. United States. URL: https://data.unicef.org/country/usa/5.

[5] Centers for Disease Control and Prevention. Infant mortality rate. URL: https://www.cdc.gov/nchs/pressroom/sosmap/infant_mortality_rates/infant_mortality.htm

[6] Ely DM, Driscoll AK. Infant mortality by selected maternal characteristics and race and Hispanic origin in the United States, 2019–2021. Natl Vital Stat Rep 2024;73(3):1-9.

[7] Statista. Real per capita gross domestic product of the United States in 2023, by state. URL: https://www.statista.com/statistics/248063/per-capita-us-real-gross-domestic-product-gdp-by-state/.

[8] World Population Review. Black population by state 2024. URL: https://worldpopulationreview.com/state-rankings/black-population-by-state.

[9] National Center for Education Statistics. Indicator 4 snapshot: Children living in poverty for racial/ethnic subgroups. URL: https://nces.ed.gov/programs/raceindicators/indicator_rads.asp#:~:text=The%20percentages%20of%20children%20living,and%20Asian%20children%20(11%20percent.

[10] Wolf ER, Rivara FP, Orr CJ, Sen A, Chapman DA, Woolf SH. Racial and ethnic disparities in all-cause and cause-specific mortality among US youth. JAMA 2024;331(20):1732-40.

[11] Braudt DB, Lawrence EM, Tilstra AM, Rogers RG, Hummer RA. Family socioeconomic status and early life mortality risk in the United States. Matern Child Health 2019;23(10):1382-91.

[12] Harms, M.B., Garrett-Ruffin, S.D. Disrupting links between poverty, chronic stress, and educational inequality. NPJ Sci Learn 2023;8(1):50.

[13] Hughes M, Tucker W. Poverty as an adverse childhood experience. NC Med J 2018;79(2):124-6.

[14] Hauptman M, Rogers ML, Scarpaci M, Morin B, Vivier PM. Neighborhood disparities and the burden of lead poisoning. Pediatr Res 2023;94:826–36.

[15] Louisias M, Phipatanakul W. Managing asthma in low-income, underrepresented minority, and other disadvantaged pediatric populations: Closing the gap. Curr Allergy Asthma Rep 2017;17(10):68.

[16] Maguire-Jack K, Font S, Dillard R, Dvalishvili D, Barnhart S. Neighborhood poverty and adverse childhood experiences over the first 15 years of life. Int J Child Maltreat 2021;4:93–114.

[17] Min J, Xue H, Wang Y. Association between household poverty dynamics and childhood overweight risk and health behaviours in the United States: A 8-year nationally representative longitudinal study of 16,800 children. Pediatr Obes 2018;13(10):590-7.

[18] Ridley M, Rao G, Schilbach F, Patel V. Poverty, depression, and anxiety: Causal evidence and mechanisms. Science 2020;370(6522):eaay0214. Erratum in: Science 2024;383(6689):eadp1916.

[19] National Center for Education Statistics. Trends in high school dropout and completion rates in the United States. URL: https://nces.ed.gov/programs/dropout/intro.asp.

[20] The Commonwealth Institute. Unequal opportunities: Fewer resources, worse outcomes for students in schools with concentrated poverty. URL: https://thecommonwealthinstitute.org/tci_research/unequal-opportunities-fewer-resources-worse-outcomes-for-students-in-schools-with-concentrated-poverty/.

[21] Hodgkinson S, Godoy L, Beers LS, Lewin A. Improving mental health access for low-income children and families in the primary care setting. Pediatrics 2017;139(1):e20151175.

[22] Manhica H, Straatmann VS, Lundin A, Agardh E, Danielsson AK. Association between poverty exposure during childhood and adolescence, and drug use disorders and drug-related crimes later in life. Addiction 2021;116(7):1747-56.

[23] Garwood SK, Lara G, Melissa J-R, Katie P, Brett D. More than poverty—Teen pregnancy risk and reports of child abuse reports and neglect. J Adolesc Health 2015;57(2):164-8.

[24] Chen, V.CH., Lee, C.TC., Wu, SI. Gossop M. Neurobehavioral disorders among children born to mothers exposed to illicit substances during pregnancy. BMC Med 2024;22:581.

[25] Break the Cycle of Health Disparities. URL: https://www.breakthecycleprogram.org/btcprogram.

Section one: Break the Cycle

Chapter 2

Examining the impact of adverse childhood experiences on educational outcomes of students with an emotional behavior disorder

Nicole Houston, BS, Med[*]
and Miles Anthony Irving, PhD
Department of Learning Sciences, College of Education and Human Development, Georgia State University, Atlanta, Georgia, United States of America

The impact of multiple adverse childhood experiences (ACEs) on a child's health and development is well known. In the field of education, ACEs have been studied to help understand students with problematic internalizing and externalizing behaviors. To date, research has not explored the association and impact of ACEs among students who qualify to receive additional school supports through individualized education plan (IEP) in the category of emotional behavior disorder (EBD). Among all disability subgroups identified in the school setting, students with EBD experience the most negative behavioral, educational and long-term outcomes while in school and after graduation. Due to systemically inequitable policies impacting minority communities, Black children are disproportionately identified as having EBD, as well as disproportionately experiencing multiple ACEs. We undertook a literature review to summarize prior research assessing behavioral, educational, and long-term outcomes of students with ACEs and students with EBD separately and explore the relationship between experiences and outcomes of children experiencing multiple ACEs and students with EBD. Our findings reveal many overlapping outcomes in the areas of

[*] Corresponding Author's E-mail: nicolehouston631@gmail.com

In: Neighborhoods: Impact on Child Health and Development
Editors: I Leslie Rubin and Joav Merrick
ISBN: 979-8-89530-834-9

education and adult health outcomes. Future research to study the relationships between ACEs and EBD is recommended for communities and schools to provide adequate resources to students who have significant behavioral challenges, especially Black students who are disproportionately affected by ACEs and disproportionately represented by EBD. Such research and resource development could serve to help break the cycle of racial disparities and inequities that impact educational performance and postsecondary outcomes, to provide the students with a promising future.

Introduction

Children are vulnerable to challenging socioeconomic and environmental influences that can affect their physical and behavioral well-being. Adverse childhood experiences (ACEs) is a term that encompasses many environmental and social challenges that children may be exposed to in their early years of life. ACEs have been studied across multiple disciplines, particularly in health and human development. The first study on ACEs, reported in 1989, administered a questionnaire to adults who received a physical examination within the year from Kaiser Permanente's San Diego-based health clinic. The questionnaire grouped the participants' past experiences into seven categories of adverse childhood experiences: psychological abuse, physical abuse, sexual abuse; violence against the mother; a substance abuser who lived in the home; someone in the home who was mentally ill or suicidal; or someone in the family who was imprisoned (1). Subsequent studies extended the categories of ACEs to include divorce or separation, physical neglect, emotional neglect, and family dysfunction (2), as well as economic hardship, and racial mistreatment (3).

While children who experience one or two ACEs may have negative health outcomes, a child who is exposed to multiple ACEs is at a far greater risk for negative health outcomes (1-3). The cumulative risk model is the most common model used to examine how an increasing number of co-occurring risk factors, in the form of multiple ACEs, are more likely to negatively affect child health and development (4). The understanding of ACEs provides insight into how links between co-occurring traumatic events impact the physical, emotional, and mental well-being of children as they grow into adults.

Children who experience multiple traumatic events may have difficulty recognizing, expressing, and understanding how their emotional reactions to their past experiences have shaped their tendency to display more aggressive and reactive behavior (2). High occurrences of ACEs in children have been linked to low academic performance and externalizing behaviors, including violence (5). Students who experienced three or more ACEs were more likely to demonstrate poor school attendance, and failure to meet grade-level standards, regardless of disability status. Students with three or more reported ACEs were four to five times more likely to have behavioral challenges compared to students with no reported exposure to ACEs (6). Children who had three or more ACEs were likely to have a four-fold increased likelihood of experiencing either internalized or externalized problematic behaviors (7). These externalized and internalized behaviors can manifest in the school setting to the degree that warrants special attention and initiates a process towards increased supports and possibly special education services.

Understanding emotional behavior disorder

In the school setting, emotional behavior disorder (EBD) is a special education category that acknowledges a student's behavior's impact on educational learning (8). Students who qualify for the label of EBD must display behaviors observed in the classroom that impede their learning. For a student to qualify for special education services under the category of EBD in the state of Georgia, they must meet certain criteria in one or more identified areas based on frequency, duration, and intensity of the problematic behaviors. These behaviors include: the inability to maintain interpersonal relationships; the inability to learn that cannot be adequately explained intellectually or because of sensory or health-related factors; chronic displays of inappropriate behavior or feelings under normal conditions; pervasive moods of unhappiness or depression; or the tendency to display physical symptoms, pains, or fears associated with personal or school problems. Students with EBD are characterized with demonstrating "inappropriate behavior or feelings under normal conditions, as well as pervasive moods of unhappiness or depression" which have an educational impact (8). Before considering whether a student qualifies for special education services or meets the criteria for EBD, students receive instruction and support in the general education setting from a general education teacher.

Schools employ various support methods to address students' academic and behavioral needs before determining if they have EBD, which would qualify them for special education services. Students receive tiered level supports, as needed, that increase in intensity and frequency towards grade-level curriculum. This multi-tiered system, called response to intervention (RTI), is designed to provide additional supports to students in the general education setting before considering special education services. All students, regardless of demographics or abilities, are entitled to receive high-quality instruction, also known as ‘tier 1 classroom instruction’, to support academic and behavioral growth. Students who do not respond to tier 1 classroom instruction in the regular classroom setting can receive additional support through tier 2 and tier 3 instruction, which increases the use of educational strategies through small group or one-on-one support settings, respectively. Before receiving a diagnosis of an EBD, students receive various levels of support using tier 2 and 3 instruction to exclude the possibility that their lack of learning is a result of inadequate instruction or lack of cognitive ability (9).

Multi-tier student supports (MTSS) or response to intervention (RTI) models suggest that about 80 percent of the school’s population should be able to learn and access grade-level curriculum with tier 1 instruction (10). Due to structural and systemic inequities, underperforming schools are more likely to be situated in low-income communities with a majority Black student population, where many students do not enter school with academic readiness skills and struggle to achieve grade-level expectations (11). When a majority of students at a school fail to meet grade level expectations, following the tiered model for supports with fidelity becomes challenging since more than the recommended percentage of students may require more intensive supports. This suggests that schools situated in low-income communities require an increased need for tier 1 supports rather than an increased need for special education services which can lead to misplacement and overrepresentation. Due to factors that are often more prevalent in low-income environments, it is vital for tier 1 supports to be conducive to the learning needs of the students in low-income communities for tiered supports to be effective.

Students with EBD require and receive more school support, including counseling, functional behavior assessments (FBA), and additional support in the general education classroom compared to students with other disability categories and students without a documented disability (12). An FBA is typically conducted before qualifying for services and attempts to determine the triggers of problematic behaviors displayed by the student in the school setting. Examples of triggers identified through an FBA include setting, time of day, being prompted to engage in a task, and/or being denied the opportunity for a task. The FBA is used to develop a behavior intervention plan (BIP) to address problematic behaviors. Students are explicitly taught coping strategies and receive consequences to decrease problematic behaviors and increase desired behaviors. In addition to an FBA, rating scales are distributed to parents and teachers to evaluate observable behaviors in various contexts, such as home and school, aiming to pinpoint clinically significant problematic behaviors. However, they may fall short of capturing the influence of past and present experiences, such as exposure to ACEs, which can potentially result in problematic behavior.

Before finding a child eligible for special education services, the school committee considers exclusionary factors that could cause an educational impact, such as socioeconomic status (SES), culture, or adequate instruction in math and reading. Despite systematically identifying students through the RTI process to ensure all students are screened and supported adequately, demographics remain stronger predictors of students being referred for special education services than academic performance (9). For example, a Black student in a predominantly White school is more likely referred for services, even when poverty is not a factor, compared to a Black student in a predominantly Black school (9). While all students may display characteristics and tendencies of problematic behaviors, Black students are more likely to be perceived as displaying challenging behaviors and receive special education services (9). This discrepancy highlights systemic biases in addressing student behavior that must be addressed to ensure fair and equitable support for all students. This is particularly important for students who have experienced co-occurring ACEs or qualify for special education services through EBD.

Intersectionality of ACEs and EBDs on behaviors of students

Structural inequities, such as racism and lack of home ownership because of historic redlining (13), are associated with higher rates of ACEs that, in turn, inhibit students' growth intellectually, interpersonally, and emotionally (14). Furthermore, individuals experience and overcome adversity differently, in part due to differences in culture, economic status, and ethnicity. Intersectionality analyses assess the overlapping disadvantages that individuals, or groups of people, experience.

Figure 1 shows the relationship between children who are exposed to multiple ACEs and school-aged children labeled as having EBD display similar internalized and externalized behaviors (4, 7, 15-19), poor academic performance (3, 6, 20-22), and experience similar health, unemployment, economic, and criminal outcomes through adolescence and adulthood (2, 5, 14, 23-26). Because Black students are disproportionately represented in the category of EBD at higher rates (15) and experience higher levels of ACEs (2, 3, 17, 27-29), understanding the links between multiple ACEs and EBD, considering factors such as race, poverty, and academic performance, could better identify environmental and socioeconomic experiences that result in emotional instability. This could ultimately avoid labeling students with negative attributes such as "deviant" when their behaviors do not align with the norms and expectations of the school and move the conversation towards understanding how traumatic experiences have shaped their childhood behaviors and reactions, and provide counseling and other supportive strategies to improve their potential for success and thus break the cycle of health and educational disparities.

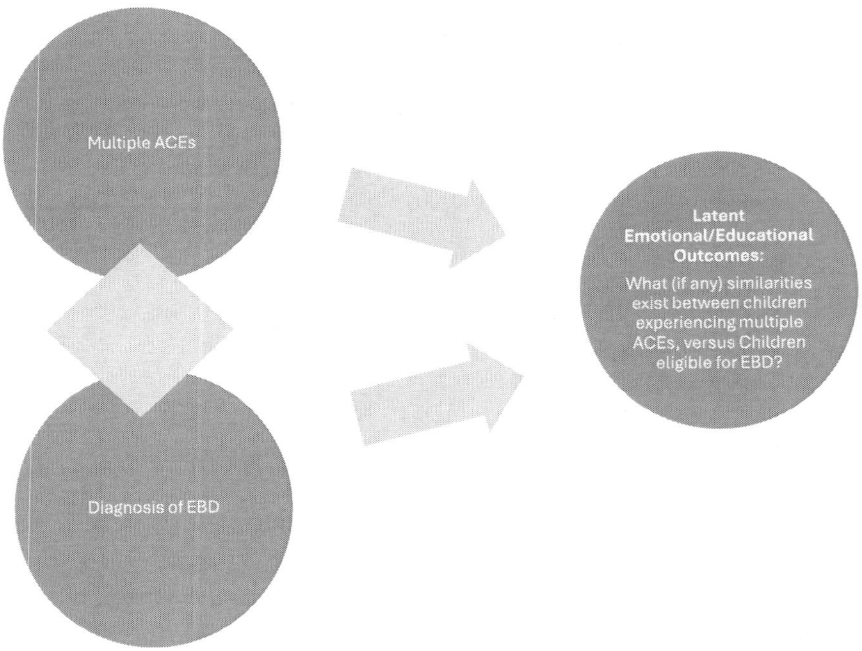

Figure 1. Relationship between ACEs, EBD and emotional/educational outcomes.

Literature gap

While research has investigated outcomes of students with ACEs and students with EBD in separate studies, to date, no research conducted in the United States has investigated the relationship or connections between ACEs and

EBD (30). This study aims to examine the educational outcomes of various racial groups that are disproportionately impacted by higher rates of ACEs and disproportionately placed in special education under the specific category of EBD. Of the research that does exist for the EBD population, limited studies examine the root causes of the behaviors displayed by students within school settings (12). The current definition of EBD suggests that students experience intensive problematic behaviors under normal conditions but does not offer a rationale for the origin students' behaviors. Behaviors observed within the school setting may not capture the actual root cause of behavior that stems from adversity in the home and community. Currently, schools do not utilize an assessment to determine the occurrence of ACEs in a child's life and therefore schools have limited context to understand and determine what causal factors might significantly impact student behaviors. Understanding the potential link between ACEs and EBD may assist school-based professionals in identifying and providing adequate tiered supports based on students' needs to be academically and socially successful in their school journey.

While the lack of special education services can lead to severely negative impacts for students with EBD, the provision of special education services has not resulted in outcomes that equalize their educational success with those of their peers (23). EBD is diagnosed along a range of emotional behaviors, and the process of identifying students is nuanced. The RTI model has limitations with the fidelity of identifying students who need tiered supports and services to thrive academically and socially. In part, problems with accurately identifying students who need increased support are due to the over-reliance on teacher expectations and the social/cultural norms of the school for students being referred for special education services (9). Understanding the root causes of students' behavior can help schools better identify the function of behaviors that severely impact learning, so the students with EBD can benefit from the levels of supports they receive. The more we understand the relationship between ACEs, problematic behavior, and EBD, the more interventions can be put in place for students negatively impacted by poverty, race, and adversity, to succeed. It is expected that this literature review will contribute to the knowledge of ACEs and EBD by exploring potential linkages between emotional and educational outcomes of students who experience multiple ACEs and who display problematic emotional behavioral disorders that are designated as EBD.

Our study

Researchers reviewed available full-text, peer-reviewed, empirical studies written in English, used quantitative measures, conducted in the United States, and published within the past fifteen years, 2012-2023. The literature review identified a few older studies occurring outside the 15-year range, which were also included to contribute to the understanding of ACEs and overrepresentation in special education (1, 15). Variations of the term ACEs were included, such as ACEs and adverse childhood experiences. ACEs were searched with additional terms, such as academics, academic achievement, academic performance, or academic success. A separate search was conducted to include a variation of ACEs and behavior outcomes. EBD was searched using the terms: EBD, emotional behavior disorder, emotional disturbance, emotion disorder and behavior disorder. These were searched with the same academic and behavior variations as the ACEs search. While no studies were found that met the criteria for being conducted in the United States, we found only one international study conducted in the Netherlands that included ACEs and EBD in the same study (30).

Studies that included children from birth through adolescence and adulthood were included in the literature review when the focus of the study was related to behavioral and academic outcomes. Few studies were found that included descriptive statistics about race, which were noted when that information was available. Studies assessing educational impact were identified through the title and abstract. Articles that discussed mental health were included when the focus of the article examined educational, post-secondary, and adult outcomes. Because the focus of this review examines the impact of ACEs on educational and emotional outcomes, the review excluded studies primarily assessing the impact ACEs have on physical health. For this review, findings on physical health are discussed secondarily among relevant articles primarily assessing educational and/or emotional outcomes. Key terms such as trauma or childhood trauma were not included, as they often examine traumatic events in isolation, and not as cooccurring events, for example, divorce or substance use in the home.

Our findings

Linkages between adverse childhood experiences, poverty and race

ACEs are more likely to occur in low-income communities (2). Due to decades of systematic racism, families living in low-income communities are more likely to be Black and more likely to be referred to the child welfare system for child maltreatment (28, 29). Black children are reported to be living below the poverty level over three times more than White children (28). Black and Hispanic children are more likely to experience higher exposure to ACEs and more likely to experience specific types of ACEs, such as domestic violence, emotional abuse, and parental death (27). Black families are more likely to live in neighborhoods that experience high poverty and crime rates, further increasing exposure to ACEs. Children who are exposed to violence and criminalization are more likely to repeat similar behaviors, making it difficult to break the cycle from disadvantageous community structures (2).

Low-income households have been linked to increased risks of poor physical and mental health but are less likely to have access to high-quality health treatment for children and adults alike, and only a small percentage of individuals living in poverty who are diagnosed with mental illnesses receive treatment, and even fewer complete treatment (31). Black children disproportionally live in poverty and are at greater risk for developing mental illness, especially when experiencing poverty for extended amounts of time (31). Unfortunately, while children are expected to visit a primary care physician annually for a checkup, universal screening for mental health is not included (31).

Children living in poverty are more likely to experience chronic stress from neighborhood violence, family dysfunction, separation of family members, and substandard living conditions. Studies have linked chronic stress and low socioeconomic status to poor neurobiological functioning, specifically affecting emotional regulation, and are more likely to experience mood dysregulation including anxiety, depression, and aggression (24). Children living in poverty, and in unsafe neighborhoods were more likely to develop anxiety or depression (24). Children's living arrangements are associated with social functioning, for example, children living with a single parent are more likely to develop anxiety or depression (32). Increased exposure to negative environmental factors that lead to anxiety and depression, can result in children displaying various levels of internalizing and externalizing behaviors.

Link between ACEs, internalizing and externalizing behaviors

Individuals who have experienced multiple ACEs are more likely to have negative health, psychological, and academic outcomes, in addition to higher engagement in criminal activity. Experiencing multiple ACEs can result in increased display of more internalized and externalized behaviors (16, 17) such as anxiety, depression, and/ or conduct disorders (2, 5, 14). These factors can play a role for adults impacted by ACEs to function and earn a stable income. Anderson et al. found when mediating for income, SES was an important contextual factor in predicting the likelihood of exposure to ACEs and in parental relationships with their children, regardless of race, gender, and marital status (16). While lower SES was associated with both internalized and externalized behaviors, a higher number of ACEs were associated with problematic behaviors in adolescents. These behaviors included hostility, aggressiveness, oppositional behavior, anxiety, and depression, particularly among children lacking adequate closeness and support. Having a supportive parent or caregiver was found to alleviate the impact of physical abuse and perceived financial insecurity on adolescents and lessened problematic behaviors. These supportive buffers may explain why not all children who experience multiple ACEs are prone to adverse behaviors, poor academic performance, and/or negative adult outcomes (16).

ACEs are more prevalent in vulnerable families, such as single parents, low income, and low education attainment, and among Black and Hispanic children. Black students, specifically those whose mothers had a high school level education or less, were more likely to be exposed to multiple ACEs compared to their White peers (17). Hunt et al. used the longitudinal dataset from the Fragile Families and Child Wellbeing Study to examine behavior patterns for non-white students at the age of 9 and those whose families were of low socioeconomic status and found that children with greater ACEs exposure were more likely to develop an attention deficit hyperactive disorder (ADHD) (17). Additionally, parent anxiety or depression consistently predicted externalizing behaviors, internalizing behaviors, and ADHD in their children (17).

Adolescents were less likely to exhibit externalizing behaviors when raised by at least one caregiver with a supportive parenting style, even when exposed to higher levels of ACEs (16). The impacts of ACEs on childhood behaviors may also be mitigated by neighborhood supports. A review of the relationship between ACEs, mental disorders, and neighborhood support from a sample of 6 to 17-year-old children using the National Survey of Children's

Health dataset, looked at four mental disorders: anxiety, depression, ADHD, and behavior problems (18). Neighborhood support was categorized as excellent, high, medium, and low based on a four-point Likert scale measuring individuals' perception of the following statements: neighbors help one another out, watch out for each other's child, and know where to go for help in the community. Results concluded that children and adolescents with three or more ACEs experienced the highest rates of having at least one of the four mental disorders and were more likely to have multiple mental disorders. Children and adolescents who rated their neighborhood as having low support experienced the highest rates of mental disorders, however, when children perceived their neighborhood as supportive, the rates of mental disorders were reduced (18). Students who experienced multiple ACEs or have been labeled with EBD, underperform academically compared to their peers who reported only experiencing one ACE (20, 21), or of any other disability subgroup (12). Additionally, students who had multiple ACEs and students with a special education label of EBD experience overlapping educational outcomes and latent outcomes in adulthood.

Educational outcomes: ACES

Children who experience four or more cumulative ACEs are more likely to have difficulties in the school setting with chronic absenteeism, lack of engagement in school, and are more likely to repeat a grade level (3). These students are also at higher risk of dropping out of school when they struggle to perform at grade level and experience a lack of academic success (3). Specific ACEs related to family dysfunction, living in poverty, and high rates of neighborhood crime are contributing factors to student attendance and performing poorly in school, and can also be factors predicting low parent involvement (3). While attendance, engagement, and retention have been found to be negatively impacted by ACEs, multiple ACEs have also been found to have a negative impact on specific critical skills for, learning and academic skills, such as self-regulation, task engagement math, language, and literacy (20). In addition, negative correlations have been found between students who experience multiple ACEs and their language and attention skills, social skills, and aggressiveness (20).

It has been well established that ACEs during early childhood is a risk factor for poor academic achievement and problematic behaviors that contribute to the achievement gap between Black and White students (21).

Students experiencing as many as five or more ACEs are more likely to encounter academic barriers preventing them from completing college (22). Students enrolled in college who experienced five or more childhood ACEs are more likely to engage in drinking that impedes their academic success, have family matters that distract them from their academics, and develop health issues or sustain injuries making it difficult to study or attend class. In addition, students with five or more ACEs were more likely to meet the criteria for depression and have a documented or suspected learning difficulty, qualifying them for special education service (22).

EBD (emotional behavior disorder)

Students with EBD should receive special education services to support their individual behavioral and educational needs. While ten to twenty percent of school-aged children experience emotional and behavioral problems that are supported through mental health services, significantly fewer students receive special education services to support their emotional and behavioral concerns (12).

Hetrick et al. (12) examined academic and behavioral functioning among students with emotional and behavioral needs looking at different school-based supports based on the student's disability and found that discipline rates and demographic variables were predictors for special education services. Students were identified before receiving special education services in the categories of specific learning disabilities (SLD), EBD, other health impaired (OHI), such as ADHD, or not receiving any special education services. Parents completed a behavior rating scale to screen for students' social, emotional, or behavior impairments. Parents also completed a demographic questionnaire to provide information related to gender, socio-economic status, ethnicity, and noted which biological parents lived within the same home as the child. Students completed behavior rating scales to identify symptoms of anxiety and depression. In addition, students were administered an achievement test and were asked about the school-based services they were receiving.

Similar to the research found with ACEs, they found a statistically significant difference in lower academic functionality, broad reading and broad math, between students with a specific learning disability and all other groups. However, no groups displayed significant differences in behavior functionality when comparing parents' or students' results of the behavior rating scales.

While students with EBD were more likely to receive supports in and outside of the classroom, compared to students with no disability or only a learning disability, students with EBD received statistically higher office discipline referrals and in-school suspension rates than all other students. There was no statistical difference in the rate of office discipline referrals or in school suspension between students with EBD and other categories addressing behavior, another special education service category that identifies inhibiting behaviors such as attention and impulsivity. Findings were consistent across several studies related to disciplinary infractions for students requiring behavioral support (12, 23).

Health behaviors

There are strong links between multiple ACEs and poor health outcomes (1). While health is not the focus of this literature review, it is important to note that students with ACEs experience negative health outcomes that negatively impact school performance (22) and students with EBD are more likely to experience poor health and engage in risky behavior that adversely impacts their health. According to the NLTS-2 substance abuse study that surveyed 18-21-year-old youths receiving special education services, students with EBD were more likely to smoke cigarettes daily, drink alcohol, use marijuana, and use other illegal drugs compared to any other disability category (26). Similar outcomes have been found for students who experience multiple ACEs (1, 21). Poor health behaviors may contribute to higher rates of absenteeism and poor performance at school, due to doctors' appointments, sick days taken at home, lethargy, and low attention, contributing to poor academic performance that leads to less educational opportunities in the future.

Latent outcomes in school-age adolescents through adulthood: ACEs

While most individuals experience at least one ACE throughout childhood, cumulative experiences are more likely to have latent impacts through adulthood. It is important to note that ACE measurement scales record the number of ACEs an individual reports but do not differentiate among the duration and intensity of the event, or the levels of caregivers and social supports available. This could explain in part why individuals with the same number of ACE occurrences do not have the same type of outcomes through adolescence and adulthood. Additionally, individuals experiencing stability and love as buffers throughout childhood may not be as adversely impacted by ACEs as others lacking such support (16).

ACEs have been found to have latent effects on increasing the likelihood of engagement in risky behaviors (14). Researchers who examined the relationship between ACEs and juvenile offenders who commit serious, violent, and chronic crimes, have proposed using an ACE scale as an early predictor of youth at risk for committing serious, violent, and chronic offenders as young adults (2). Results have shown a greater number of ACEs were experienced by serious, violent, and chronic offenders compared to one-time non-violent offenders, and the youth who engage in serious and violent crimes who had experienced higher rates of ACEs, continue to display problematic behaviors and risky behaviors throughout adulthood (2).

Hicks and Smith-Darden (19) analyzed the links between cumulative ACEs and psychological distress, substance abuse, and delinquency among Black youth. Their research incorporated a longitudinal study with 265 participants, ages 7-13 years, from six school districts in Southeast Michigan, utilizing the lens of social learning theory to explain how victimization and witnessing harm against social norms can lead to externalized behaviors in later life. They used the original ACEs scale to survey students annually for four years. While exposure to multiple ACEs can lead to substance abuse and delinquency, these outcomes can be exacerbated by distress. They concluded that the more ACEs an individual experiences, the more likely that individual will display problematic behaviors, demonstrate poor academic achievement, and experience negative outcomes in adulthood (19).

EBD (emotional behavior disorder)

Students who have been labeled with EBD are more likely to engage in risky behaviors that impact their health and/or engage in criminal activity (23). Freeman et al. (23) found consistently poor primary, secondary, and post-secondary educational outcomes for students with EBD who are also more likely to be suspended from school; receive disciplinary infractions for drugs, weapons, and causing bodily injury; be served in an alternative setting separate from their nondisabled peers, which has a negative academic impact on their ability to perform at a comparable level to their same-aged peers and contributes to dropping out of high school. In addition, students with EBD are also more likely to be arrested and incarcerated than their peers with a different disability or those without a disability.

The National Longitudinal Transition Study-2 (NLTS-2) conducted an 8-year follow-up interview and questionnaire with students, parents, teachers, and other school staff to evaluate the experiences, characteristics, and outcomes of students who received special education services (26). The nationally representative sample consisted of students who were receiving special education services no later than grade 7 and were between the ages of 13-16 years at the start of the study. According to the NLTS-2, at least 75 percent of students with EBD were involved with the criminal justice system within the first eight years after leaving high school, being stopped by police, arrested, staying overnight in jail, and being on probation. While students with EBD were as likely as their peers with other disabilities to enroll in post-secondary schooling, they earned fewer credits while enrolled and were less likely to complete post-secondary schooling. For employment, students with EBD were likely to gain employment after high school but were more likely to get fired or laid off compared to other disability categories, except for individuals with an intellectual disability. Individuals with EBD were the most likely to be unemployed at the time of the interview. Compared to other disability categories, except for individuals with an intellectual disability, students with EBD were more likely to work in an entry-level position in food service. Individuals with EBD were less likely to have savings accounts and likely to earn $25,000 or less, more likely to have had a child within eight years of high school, more likely to live in poverty, and more likely to participate in negative community activities, defined by fighting and carrying a weapon (26).

In a survey of repeat juvenile offenders, 90 percent of repeat juvenile offenders reported they had experienced multiple ACEs (2). Students with EBD are more likely to be arrested and incarcerated compared to other disability subgroups and their non-disabled peers (26). Individuals who have reported multiple ACEs (2, 19) and students with EBD (7) are more likely to be suspended and receive disciplinary infractions in school. Despite students with EBD receiving additional services, they continue to demonstrate an increased need to have access to the same opportunities as their non-disabled peers.

Discussion

Poverty has a negative impact on the foundation of communities and contributes to emotional stress that in turn, negatively impacts academic success. Lower academic success leads to a higher chance of dropping out of school, contributing to fewer job opportunities and lower income to support sustainable healthy living conditions, and perpetuates the cycle of poverty and consequently, health disparities. Black children are most impacted as they are more likely to live in impoverished communities, experience ACEs, and emotional stressors that are associated with internalizing and externalizing behaviors such as anxiety, depression, and aggression. Schools serving students in impoverished communities who are at greater risk for multiple ACEs, should be prepared to offer substantial and specific supports to reduce the likelihood of disadvantageous outcomes and meet students' needs throughout their educational careers. Taking a 'whole child' approach by addressing the needs of the child beyond the classroom and reducing the intensity of the impacts of systemic inequities, can in turn, reduce the negative impact of ACEs at the individual, family, and community level. This approach needs to be instituted for children as young as possible, preferably in the elementary school grades, to have a greater impact on the prevention of the potentially destructive outcomes related to ACEs.

It is important to note that what researchers have classified as ACEs may differ from what may be perceived by the youth as adverse. For example, in one study, adolescents defined the following as adverse experiences: family relationships, community stressors, personal victimization, economic hardship, peer relationships, discrimination, school, health, child welfare/juvenile justice, and media/technology (33). Family relationships were the highest reported domain for stressors and was defined by specific events: family members abusing alcohol and drugs, lack of love and support in the family, single-parent homes, death and illness of family members, violence in the home, poor parenting and lack of guidance, criminal activity by family members, having to take on adult responsibilities, and violent victimization of family members by individuals outside of the home. Negative adult behavior in the neighborhood, classified as a community stressor, was the most experienced adversity. Understanding what children perceive as stressors and how they feel impacted by the identified stressors, could provide insight into specific interventions and supports that may be beneficial at the individual, family, and community level.

Black children encounter increased emotional stress due to intergenerational disadvantages which perpetuate cycles of economic hardship and reduced opportunities for upward mobility. When students struggle to successfully attain an education, the impacts of poverty can be further exacerbated, continuing a cycle of poverty, inequities and disadvantageous outcomes. Schools may further perpetuate inequities by misidentifying the needs of students and failing to provide adequate supports for students who are experiencing adversity that contribute to their lack of academic and social success. By acknowledging and addressing the adversities that children experience outside of school that have an impact on student learning while in school, schools could counterbalance racial disparities among students.

Strategies for breaking the cycle

School leaders have the authority to identify professional development needs to build capacity within schools, so that school teachers and staff members can be prepared, equipped and sensitive to individual student situations, especially for the students who are at risk for EBD. School leaders should also evaluate the effectiveness of their current social and emotional learning (SEL) programs that promote healthy social and emotional development. Currently, SEL supports rely on teachers for implementation. However, more schools need to partner with mental health agencies to provide mental health support to students during the school day. Additionally, school leaders should collaborate with therapists and other student support services staff to distribute ACE surveys to all students, to identify students who would benefit from additional community resources and school-based support, especially at the younger ages. School-based support includes trauma-informed practices, such as professional development for staff and the implementation of restorative practices, allowing schools to be safe havens for students who have experienced trauma, by providing compassion and being resilience-oriented (34). One of the greatest benefits of trauma-informed practices is creating awareness around the latent impact that co-occurring adversities have on an individual, so adults who care for children are more sensitive to the child's environment, and to positive environmental changes that will help a child to thrive (35).

In addition to including more SEL and therapy services provided by a licensed professional during the school day, policymakers should consider the flexibility that schools need to incorporate services that will prevent students from missing instruction during the school day and reduce the risk of falling further behind. For example, schools can develop resources to provide internet access with more virtual learning days, and/or intervention blocks embedded during the day. Difficulty in having parent-teacher conferences during the day could be a lack of child-care and participation, especially for single-parent households, therefore, flexible times, possibly outside of typical school hours, could be allocated for routine parent-teacher conferences to build stronger relationships between students, parents, and school staff. Another option can be for school staff to routinely visit communities and meet with community members and families in neighborhoods instead of community members and families commuting to schools. Increasing access to school personnel and resources offered by the school could build the initial relationship for families who are perceived to be less involved but who have barriers to physically attending school events. The collective effort and collaboration between communities and schools could strengthen the support students may not otherwise experience. Including the community as a part of the solution allows for a positive environment where individuals can build supportive relationships and thrive rather than function in survival mode to withstand adversities. Community resiliency levels can also determine which intervention programs should be implemented in the community and may be best supported and maintained by the community (36).

Promoting resilience at the individual, family, and community level can reduce the negative impact of ACEs. There is an inverse correlation between measures of resiliency and mental health outcomes, such as ADHD, anxiety, and depression. Children with four or more ACE occurrences were more likely to develop mental health concerns, problematic behaviors, poor school performance, and negative work outcomes, compared to children with less than four. However, resiliency can be a mitigating factor on community-wide levels of mental health, problem behaviors, and school/ work outcomes when controlling for the number of ACEs, low-income status, and race (32, 36).

Key components of resiliency in children explore levels of problem-solving skills, self-regulation, and relationships with caring adults compared to key components of resiliency in adults that explore self-efficacy, secure attachment, emotional support, effective decision-making, and control of one's thoughts and feelings. Resiliency in childhood can lead to improving the child's mental health with persistence of resiliency into adulthood. Problem-solving skills are linked to cognitive and social development, and children who learn skills to self-regulate can better cope with stress by being able to express their feelings and control their behavior. As a result, social skills can be improved which could, in turn, have a positive impact on educational outcomes. Experiencing academic success could lead to more positive economic outcomes later in life, such as higher-income employment options. Thus, even though students who are exposed to ACEs are more likely to be negatively impacted in other aspects of their lives and perpetuate an intergenerational cycle of poverty, we posit that this cycle can be mediated at the individual, family, and community level to break the cycle of children's health disparities.

Strengths and limitations

This literature review successfully identified commonalities and onnections between children who had ACEs and school-aged children identified with EBD. In addition, the literature review suggested how addressing the root causes of students with EBD can be mitigated through the effective incorporation of tier 1 interventions within the school setting and help promote healthy development for all children and improve their outcomes, regardless of special education status. A limitation is that additional research and empirical evidence is needed to determine the strength of these associations, as, to date, only one empirical study conducted in the Netherlands investigated the educational, emotional, and mental health outcomes of students with EBD who also experienced ACEs (30).

Next steps in research

This literature review has highlighted the similarity in experiences and outcomes among students experiencing multiple ACEs and those diagnosed with EBD. Previous studies have examined the impact of ACEs on physical health, mental health, internalized and externalized behaviors, students with conduct disorders, and juvenile delinquency, yet screening for ACEs is currently not performed among students who demonstrate frequent problematic emotional behaviors. Given that students with EBD experience more unfavorable academic and nonacademic life outcomes compared to their peers, the effectiveness of the current supports students with EBD are receiving should be reconsidered and revised. Future research should further explore the links between students with cumulative ACEs and EBD, to redefine the eligibility process for an EBD designation and better identify interventions for expected responses towards reducing further negative and challenging experiences and improving performance, resilience, and outcome. Establishing a relationship between multiple ACEs and behaviors that meet definitions for EBD, could encourage stronger supports in the school system for the children in need, and help to improve their academic and long-term outcomes.

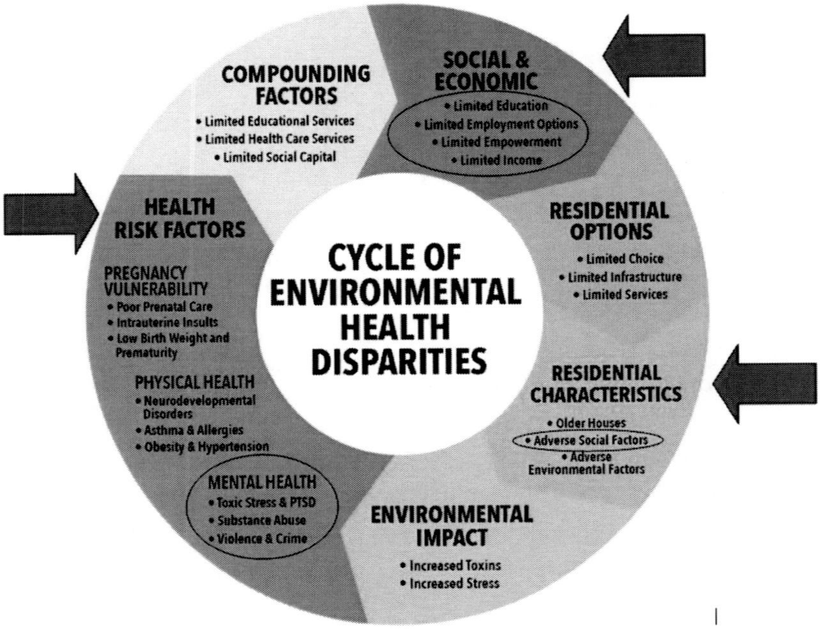

Figure 2. Breaking the cycle of children's health disparities.

Conclusion

This review provides evidence for the important connection and associations between students who have multiple ACEs and EBD, and can be informative for school leaders, student support services, and policymakers to develop programs to support these vulnerable students and improve their academic and social outcomes. Schools have access to students from childhood through young adulthood and can serve as a resource not only for academics, but also for behavior support, psychological health, post-secondary options, and more. The primary focus for students in school is to learn, and learning is associated with self-efficacy, self-regulation, and attention, which can be diminished by the impacts of adversity. Therefore, it is incumbent on the school to identify students at risk for disorders of learning and behavior, particularly for the potential designation of EBD, and to develop strategies to address their psychological, emotional and social needs so that they can take full advantage of their educational opportunities and succeed academically. Providing specific supports that are accessible to students, and that address the causal nature of their distress, without assigning potentially negative labels could help improve future outcomes for individuals who have experienced multiple ACEs and are impacted by poverty and racial mistreatment, thereby breaking the cycle of children's health disparities and improving their chances for good health and social and economic success (figure 2).

Acknowledgements

The preparation for this manuscript was supported by Break the Cycle of Health Disparities Program along with Dr. Miles Irving and Dr. Ann Kruger, professors at Georgia State University. The authors have no conflicts of interest or financial relationships to disclose.

References

[1] Felitti VJ, Anda RF, Nordenberg D, Williamson DF, Spitz AM, Edwards V, et al. Relationship of childhood abuse and household dysfunction to many of the leading causes of death in adults. Am J Prev Med 1998;14(4):245–58. https://doi.org/10.1016/s0749-3797(98)00017-8.

[2] Fox, BH, Perez N, Cass E, Baglivio MT, Epps, N. Trauma changes everything: Examining the relationship between adverse childhood experiences and serious, violent and chronic juvenile offenders. Child Abuse Neglect 2015;46:163–73. https://doi.org/10.1016/j.chiabu.2015.01.011.

[3] Crouch E, Radcliff E, Hung P, Bennett K. Challenges to school success and the role of adverse childhood experiences. Acad Pediatrics 2019;19(8):899–907. https://doi.org/10.1016/j.acap.2019.08.006.

[4] Henry LM, Gracey K, Shaffer A, Ebert J, Kuhn T, Watson KH, et al. Comparison of three models of adverse childhood experiences: Associations with child and adolescent internalizing and externalizing symptoms. J Abn Psychology 2021;130(1):9–25. https://doi.org/10.1037/abn0000644.

[5] Burke NJ, Hellman JL, Scott, BG, Weems, CF, Carrion, VG. The impact of adverse childhood experiences on an urban pediatric population. Child Abuse Neglect 2011;35(6): 408–13. https://doi.org/10.1016/j.chiabu.2011.02.006.

[6] Blodgett C, Lanigan JD. The association between adverse childhood experience (ACE) and school success in elementary school children. School Psychol Quart 2018;33(1):137–46. https://doi.org/10.1037/spq0000256.

[7] Freeman PAC. Prevalence and relationship between adverse childhood experiences and child behavior among young children. Infant Ment Health J 2014;35(6):544–54. https://doi.org/10.1002/imhj.21460.

[8] Emotional and behavioral disorder. Special Education Services and Supports. URL: https://www.gadoe.org/Curriculum-Instruction-and-Assessment/Special-Education.

[9] Dever BV, Raines TC, Barclay C, Mitchell B, Kamphaus RW. Addressing disproportionality in special education using a universal screener. PsycEXTRA Dataset 2012. https://doi.org/10.7709/jnegroeducation.85.1.0059.

[10] Pullen PC, van Dijk W, Gonsalves VE, Lane HB, Ashworth KE. RTI and MTSS: Response to intervention and multi-tiered systems of support: How do they differ and how are they the same, If at all? In: Pullen PC, Kennedy MJ, eds. Handbook of response to intervention and multi-tiered systems of support. New York: Routledge, 2018:5-10.

[11] Schueler BE, West MR. Federalism, race, and the politics of turnaround: US public opinion on improving low-performing schools and districts. Educ Res 2021;51(2):122–33.

[12] Hetrick AA, Kern L, Dever BV. Comparison of educationally labeled and nonlabeled adolescents with emotional and behavioral needs. Behav Disord 2021;47(4):245–56. https://doi.org/10.1177/01987429211052917.

[13] Huang SJ, Sehgal NJ. Association of historic redlining and present-day health in Baltimore. PLoS One 2022;17(1):e0261028. https://doi.org/10.1371/journal.pone.0261028.

[14] Parnes MKF, Schwartz SEO. Adverse childhood experiences: Examining latent classes and associations with physical, psychological, and risk-related outcomes in adulthood. Child Abuse Neglect 2022;127:105562. https://doi.org/10.1016/j.chiabu.2022.105562.

[15] Cullinan D, Kauffman JM. Do race of student and race of teacher influence ratings of emotional and behavioral problem characteristics of students with emotional disturbance? Behav Disord 2005;30(4):393–402. https://doi.org/10.1177/019874290503000403.

[16] Anderson AS, Siciliano RE, Henry LM, Watson KH, Gruhn MA, Kuhn TM, et al. Adverse childhood experiences, parenting, and socioeconomic status: Associations with internalizing and externalizing symptoms in adolescence. Child Abuse Neglect 2022;125: 105493. https://doi.org/10.1016/j.chiabu.2022.105493.

[17] Hunt, TKA, Slack KS, Berger LM. Adverse childhood experiences and behavioral problems in middle childhood. Child Abuse Neglect 2017;67:391–402. https://doi.org/10.1016/j.chiabu.2016.11.005.

[18] Khanijahani A, Sualp K. Adverse childhood experiences, neighborhood support, and internalizing and externalizing mental disorders among 6–17 years old US children: Evidence from a population-based study. Commun Ment Health J 2021;58(1):166–78. https://doi.org/10.1007/s10597-021-00808-7.

[19] Hicks MR, Kernsmith, P, Smith-Darden J. The effects of adverse childhood experiences on internalizing and externalizing behaviors among black children and Youth. J Child Adolesc Trauma 2020;14(1):115–22. https://doi.org/10.1007/s40653-020-00316-y.

[20] Lipscomb ST, Hatfield B, Lewis H, Goka-Dubose E, Abshire C. Adverse childhood experiences and children's development in early care and education programs. J Appl Dev Psychol 2021;72:101218. https://doi.org/10.1016/j.appdev.2020.101218.

[21] Jimenez ME, Wade R, Lin Y, Morrow LM, Reichman NE. Adverse experiences in early childhood and kindergarten outcomes. Pediatrics 2016;137(2):e20151839. https://doi.org/10.1542/peds.2015-1839.

[22] Hinojosa R, Nguyen J, Sellers,K, Elassar, H. Barriers to college success among students that experienced adverse childhood events. J Am Coll Health 2018;67(6): 531–40. https://doi.org/10.1080/07448481.2018.1498851.

[23] Freeman J, Yell ML, Shriner JG., Katsiyannis A. Federal policy on improving outcomes for students with emotional and behavioral disorders: Past, present, and future. Behav Disord 2018;44(2):97–106. https://doi.org/10.1177/0198742918814423.

[24] Kim P, Evans GW, Angstadt M, Ho SS, Sripada CS, Swain JE, et al. Effects of childhood poverty and chronic stress on emotion regulatory brain function in adulthood. Proceed Natl Acad Sci 2013;110(46):18442-7. https://doi.org/10.1073/pnas.1308240110.

[25] Yu J. Facts from NLTS2: Substance use among young adults with disabilities. National Center for Education Statistics (NCES) Home Page. URL: https://nces.ed.gov/pubsearch/pubsinfo.asp?pubid=NCSER20083009.

[26] Newman L, Wagner M, Knokey AM, Marder C, Nagle K, Shaver D, et al. The post-high school outcomes of young adults with disabilities up to 8 years after high school. A report from the National Longitudinal Transition Study-2 (NLTS2) (NCSER 2011-3005). Menlo Park, CA: SRI International, 2011.

[27] Maguire-Jack K, Lanier P, Lombardi, B. Investigating racial differences in clusters of adverse childhood experiences. Am J Orthopsychiatry 2020;90(1):106–14. https://doi.org/10.1037/ort0000405.

[28] Drake B, Lee SM, Jonson-Reid M. Race and child maltreatment reporting: Are Blacks overrepresented? Child Youth Serv Rev 2009;31(3):309–16. https://doi.org/10.1016/j.childyouth.2008.08.00429.

[29] Landers AL, Carrese DH, Spath R. A decade in review of trends in social work literature: The link between poverty and child maltreatment in the United States. Child Welfare 2019;97(4):65–96.

[30] Offerman EC, Asselman MW, Bolling F, Helmond P, Stams, GJJ, Lindauer RJ. Prevalence of adverse childhood experiences in students with emotional and behavioral disorders in special education schools from a multi-informant

perspective. Int J Environ Res Public Health 2022;19(6):3411. https://doi.org/10.3390/ijerph19063411.

[31] Hodgkinson S, Godoy L, Beers LS, Lewin A. Improving mental health access for low-income children and families in the primary care setting. Pediatrics 2017;139(1):20151175. https://doi.org/10.1542/peds.2015-1175.

[32] Okwori G. Role of individual, family, and community resilience in moderating effects of adverse childhood experiences on mental health among children. J Dev Behav Pediatr 2022;43(7):e452-62. https://doi.org/10.1097/dbp.0000000 00000107621.

[33] Wade R, Shea JA, Rubin D, Wood J. Adverse childhood experiences of low-income urban youth. Pediatrics 2014;134(1):e13-20. https://doi.org/10.1542/peds.2013-2475.

[34] Nctsnadmin. Creating, supporting, and sustaining trauma-informed schools: A system framework. The National Child Traumatic Stress Network. URL: https://www.nctsn.org/resources/creating-supporting-and-sustaining-trauma-informed-schools-system-framework.

[35] Bateson K, McManus M, Johnson G. Understanding the use, and misuse, of adverse childhood experiences (aces) in trauma-informed policing. Police J 2019;93(2):131–45. https://doi.org/10.1177/0032258x19841409.

[36] Longhi D, Brown M, Fromm Reed S. Community-wide resilience mitigates adverse childhood experiences on adult and Youth Health, school/work, and problem behaviors. Am Psychol 2021;76(2):216–29. https://doi.org/10.1037/amp0000773.

Chapter 3

Evaluating the effectiveness of pandemic-era anti-eviction policies on children's health

Anna McPeak*
College of Law, Georgia State University, Atlanta, Georgia, United States of America

Evictions result in a myriad of health and mental problems for adults and children alike. The impacts of eviction on children include displacement, health risks, and behavioral problems. These outcomes have not been well documented, and data is thus unavailable to policymakers when making laws. In 2021, a handful of states implemented statutory changes to alleviate the pressure tenants often feel upon receiving notice of an eviction. This chapter seeks to evaluate 1) the effectiveness of statutory changes on children's health, 2) rates of tenant confidence in ability to pay rent in states that imposed these new laws and 3) whether these laws had any impact on poverty rates. Additionally, this study postulates how these laws can have impact, and findings will guide future studies of eviction impacts on children's health.

Introduction

Eviction results in devastating and longstanding impacts to individuals and their families. When a judge issues a final judgment for eviction, within a few days an eviction crew removes everything from inside the family's home, placing it on the side of the road. This process involves removing furniture, toys, and all personal belongings, including children's medicines, and birth certificates (1). When executed under court order, this process of tenant

---

* Corresponding Author's E-mail: annamcpeak@gmail.com

In: Neighborhoods: Impact on Child Health and Development
Editors: I Leslie Rubin and Joav Merrick
ISBN: 979-8-89530-834-9

dispossession and removal proceeds under the direction of the United States Marshals Service or the County Sheriff's office (2). Although case law or statutory law exists in every state against illegal evictions, or "self-help evictions," in many states, landlords can often perform a "just cause eviction" which means "landlords do not need to justify their decision to evict someone." (2). Evictions, or dispossessory actions, are typically fast-moving processes, and tenants have little power to stop them because the balance of power between landlords and tenants is unequal (3).

The impact of eviction on children is particularly profound. Abruptly removing children from the stability of a home can result in an array of health problems. Adverse Childhood Experiences, (ACEs) are potentially traumatic events that occur in childhood, between the ages of zero and 17 years, with significant adverse physical and mental health consequences, this can include experiencing homelessness or unstable housing (4). Often, children end up in worse housing after an eviction, and "poor housing can be [.........] destructive to their emotional, psychological, and behavioral health and development" (5), which include anxiety, depression, or aggressive behaviors (5).

Every year, landlords file an average 3.6 million eviction cases (6). Of those, nearly half, or roughly 1.5 million, result in eviction judgments (7). Thus, evictions are commonplace in many neighborhoods across the country. Yet the law has limited protections for tenants and provides disproportionate control and authority to landlords, especially for tenants who have fallen behind on rent (8). The law is indicative of the power imbalance, as evictions proceedings can be confusing and devastating for those tenants involved (9).

Aside from losing housing, legal papers frequently contain arcane and stilted legal jargon describing the lease agreement or sanctions the landlord is seeking. Examples of lease language include statements such as, "pursuant to the lease dated January 1, 2020, under which you hold the possession of the herein described premises…" The language employed can also be confusing, threatening dispossession by warning that "Failure to pay… will result in forfeiture of the lease and will institute a dispossessory action against you" (10). Without appropriate legal counsel, and with the notices containing obscure language, tenants often do not know what claims they should make to counter an eviction suit. A tenant can only stop an eviction with viable counterclaims; for example, counterclaims regarding living conditions, which are futile when the reason for the eviction is lack of rent payments (9, 11). Additionally, suits have two parts to them: the dispossessory (or eviction), and a money judgment, (or what the tenant owes). Therefore, even if the eviction moves forward, a tenant may be able to reduce part – or all – of the money judgment with counterclaims.

The impacts felt by children, including health risks, displacement, and behavioral problems, have not been well documented and therefore the data is not available for policymakers to consider when making laws (12). As a result, evictions have become a "quiet epidemic." Although the COVID-19 pandemic highlighted the frequency of evictions, few initiatives have been established to keep people housed (8). In 2021, however, states began implementing statutory changes that work to protect the rights of tenants. This chapter explores those laws and their effectiveness in keeping families housed, and in turn, protecting children's health. This chapter also considers how eviction prevention laws and policies can prevent evictions from occurring, alleviating one stimulus for mental health issues afflicting children, which constitute some of our country's most vulnerable populations.

Evictions disproportionately affect low-income tenants and children of color

Those at highest risk of eviction are low-income women, especially women of color, especially if they have children (13, 14). According to a 2018 report by "Housing matters," 7.9 percent of children experienced eviction by the age of 15 years (15). The disproportionate impacts of the criminal justice system on the lives of Black men parallels the disproportionate impacts of eviction through the civil justice system on the lives of black women. Black men are six times as likely to be incarcerated as white men, and black female renters are disproportionately threatened with eviction (13, 16). By some accounts, black female renters are evicted at twice the rate of white renters (17). Consider the reflection of Matthew Desmond, founder of The Eviction Lab, who stated "If incarceration had come to define the lives of men from impoverished black neighborhoods, eviction was shaping the lives of women. Poor black men were locked up. Poor black women were locked out" (18).

With this information as background, the statutory changes that started in 2021 will be evaluated and discussed through a hypothetical case study about a woman named Max. Max's story is not about a real person but instead portrays a common scenario experienced by many female tenants. Max is a woman we likely interact with on any given day. She is a mother of a child who has health difficulties. She works multiple part-time jobs to provide for her family. She may serve us our lunch, check us in at the hospital, or clean our hotel room. She juggles many work responsibilities to keep the lights on so her children can do their homework, keep the heat on so her children stay warm, and pay for groceries so her children are fed. Max, and women like her, may even need to earn money to make sure her children have the medical care and medications they need for their asthma, anxiety and depression, or the myriad of other health issues they may be facing. Max struggles financially and emotionally throughout each day.

In 2020, Max got COVID infected without paid time off or any other benefits while she is away from work. For two weeks she stays home and does not get paid. When she finally returns to work, Max scrambles to pay heating and electric bills, and to buy groceries. As a result, she falls behind on rent. Max's landlord does not accept partial payments, because where she lives doing so is like accepting full rent, so they lose their rights if they accept any money. The Georgia Court of Appeals has held that a new, quasi-contract can be created if a landlord repeatedly accepts late or irregular payments. See, e.g., Hatchett Firm, P.C. v. Atlanta Life Financial Group 358 Ga.App. 607; see also EPI-USE Systems Limited v. BI Brainz, LLC, 2022 WL 220192. Consequently, even though Max is back at work, and may be able to pay some of her rent, she ultimately falls behind and cannot catch up.

The eviction process

An eviction occurs when a landlord expels tenant(s) from the property that he or she owns. They are "landlord initiated, involuntary moves that happen to renters" (19). Princeton University's Eviction Lab describes the five stages of eviction, also known as a dispossessory action (20). Max's eviction will start when she receives an eviction notice, which is typically the first step in the eviction process. Notice is the first step of the eviction process. (21).

Eviction notices are generally issued no matter the adversity that a family, community, or country may be facing. Families in New Orleans received eviction notices in November 2005 following Hurricane Katrina, for nonpayment of rent for October and November (22). While New Orleans faced a hurricane, another city might have experienced a flood or a tornado, but, in 2020 the onset of the COVID-19 pandemic reached every city across the United States, resulting in increased and worsened eviction rates (23).

The second step in the process involves Max's landlord filing with the court to have her removed from the property (21). Max must respond to the notice she received to avoid a default judgment, which is when the court automatically grants judgment against a party if he or she fails to answer the landlord's complaint (24). Oftentimes, women in Max's situation do not know how to respond to an issued notice. They may not know how to fill out the paperwork, or how to make any counterclaims. Max has not had to deal with anything like this before, as she just received her first eviction notice.

During the third step in the eviction process, if the tenant answered the notice, the court will have a hearing (21). In Georgia, the hearing is brief because the trial court must expedite as much as is reasonably possible (21). The fourth step happens at the end of the hearing when the court issues a decision (21).

Finally, if the process plays out like it often does, the fifth step ends with eviction (21). Deputies will arrive at Max's door and begin taking everything out of her home, including her furniture, jewelry, IDs, and sensitive papers. Max will not have time to pack her medications or a change of clothes for her or her children. She will soon be looking at a curbside full of what was once her home. Importantly, her children, who may be struggling with school, friends, fitting in, etc. will now be faced with a fundamental upheaval of their entire lives. The children caught in the crossfire of eviction may have to leave school, make new friends, and deal with the embarrassment they may feel of having to tell people why these events are occurring. If a child has learning disabilities, Max, and parents like her, may have to move her individual education plan (IEP) to a new school.

The impacts of evictions

Starting with the notice, a tenant's access to stable housing begins to diminish; the further the eviction process proceeds, the closer a family gets to facing a dispossessory action and the further away the tenant gets from access to stable housing (25). Judge's must comply with the law, and if the law requires a tenant be removed from the property, the judges do not have authority to allow a tenant to stay despite obvious adverse consequences (26). Additionally, evicted tenants are less likely to find stable housing after an eviction (27).

Landlord tenant law is governed by each state; thus, evictions operate differently depending on where a tenant lives (28). The same five basic stages apply nationally, however, and an individual whose landlord files a notice in court can be impacted whether she is ever ejected from her home, because the filing becomes public record for seven years (29). Often, landlords can see that a potential tenant had an eviction filing and will be less likely to allow the tenant to rent at their property, even if the case was dismissed (30). Though an eviction or court record will not appear on a credit report, future landlords can see the public record (31, 32). This leaves tenants with few housing options after an eviction filing and even fewer clean, safe, and stable housing options (27).

A tenant's inability to pay rent in full remains the most common reason for eviction (19). "The majority of poor renting families spend over half of their income on housing and at least one in four dedicates over 70 percent to paying the rent and keeping the lights on" (8, 18). Families in situations like Max, where the tenant gets COVID, making any illness-related absence from work an especially poignant circumstance. However, landlords can evict tenants for a broad range of other reasons, including tenants who may be housing extra people, damage of property, causing a nuisance or disturbance, or breaking the law (19, 33). With rental housing costs increasing, many renters already live below the poverty line, and many hold jobs paying hourly wages, so that falling behind on rent is a likely possibility (34, 35).

To make matters worse, evidence shows that families with children are more likely to be evicted than households without children (14). Emily Benfer, Visiting Research Collaborator at The Eviction Lab, explains:

> [D]espite the Fair Housing Act's prohibition of discrimination on the basis of familial status, families with children are three times more likely to be evicted than other households. Families of children born with adverse birth outcomes are substantially more likely to be evicted in the first 5 years of their child's life. The highest risk of eviction falls among families with Black children, who are nearly twice as likely as white children to be evicted. (14).

Children who face an increased risk of eviction, also face a higher risk of adverse health outcomes (36, 37). Mental illness is a concern for all children, but, as discussed earlier, evicted households are more likely to live in poor quality housing which puts children at an increased risk of depression, anxiety, and behavioral problems (5). Confronting this data means state government should implement policies that prevent evictions and provide stable housing for children.

Eviction cases are most concentrated in the Southeastern region of the country in large part because state-level landlord-tenant legal policy in this region is permissive of landlords filing evictions; in other words, landlords file evictions at a much higher frequency in the Southeast than anywhere else in the country (7).

Eviction often causes families to move to a new neighborhood or school district (38). Evicted individuals struggle to find jobs, and adults and children alike are exposed to food insecurity, anxiety, and depression and increased health risks. (38). For a child, eviction means the loss of home, neighborhoods, and school, leading to increased poverty, limited resources, which can lead to mental illness, including depression and emotional trauma, which linger into adulthood (39). The accumulation of these multiple intersecting ACEs, compounded by the eviction process, results in poor health as an adult (39). Addressing any one of them could help break the cycle of adverse outcomes to children and families that are caused by evictions (see figure 1).

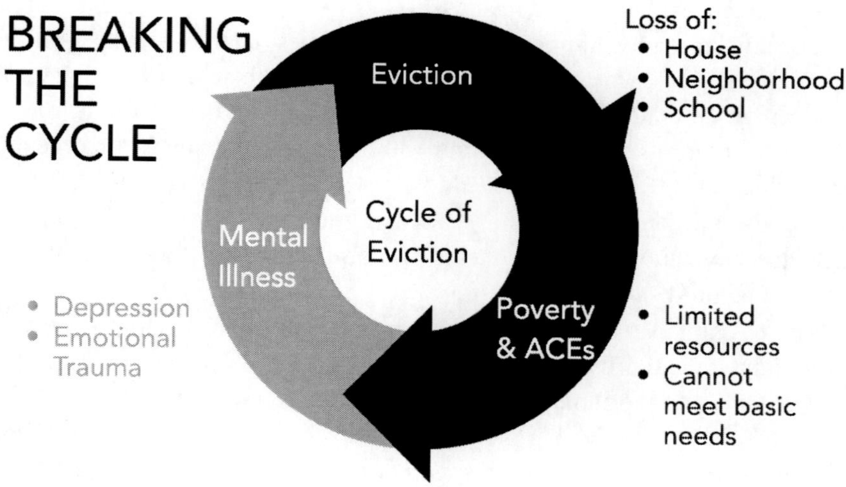

Figure 1. Breaking the cycle.

Statutory changes can help, and the laws discussed in this review were crafted and calibrated to promote more stable living arrangements for tenants, while also considering landlord's rights. Given the newness of such laws, the research performed and explained below is inconclusive. To be certain, studies reassessing and researching the impact of such statutory changes, especially on children, will be required in subsequent years.

Eviction moratoriums: A statutory change

During the COVID-19 pandemic, the government imposed various eviction moratoriums (40, 41). Moratoriums are temporary forced suspensions of an activity that stay in place until future considerations warrant the activity to resume. Effectively, moratoriums allow an otherwise legal activity to stop while a hardship endures. The CARES Act eviction moratorium began on March 27, 2020, and ended on July 24, 2020 (40). The moratorium ordered landlords not to evict tenants for lack of rent because of the COVID-19 pandemic (40).

Soon after the CARES Act moratorium ended, the Center for Disease Control and Prevention (CDC) imposed a nationwide, temporary moratorium on residential evictions for nonpayment of rent lasting from September 4, 2020, through the end of August 2021 (40, 42). Although these eviction moratoriums provided immense relief to families unable to pay rent in "staying" evictions, (meaning postponing or halting the eviction judgment), (24) neither moratorium prevented evictions altogether, though rental assistance programs provided support (40). The US Treasury's Emergency Rental Assistance (ERA) provided over $46 billion to support housing stability during the pandemic (43). The program provided over 10 million assistance payments to renters facing eviction, especially low-income and renters of color (43).

The CARES Act eviction moratorium applied only to federal properties and prohibited landlords from charging fees or penalties for unpaid rent (40, 41). The CDC moratorium applied only to renters who met income and other eligibility criteria. (40). Under the CARES Act, covered individuals could not be forced to vacate, and landlords could not file notices until 30 days after the moratorium ended (40). The CDC moratorium, on the other hand, though extended numerous times, did not address notices to vacate (40). Neither moratorium forgave unpaid rent amounts (40).

These moratoriums, though imperfect, provided a great amount of relief for tenants. According to Eviction Lab, between eviction moratoriums and rental assistance, more than a million US households avoided losing their home during the pandemic, and eviction filings were around 50% below average (44, 45). An important note about the CDC eviction moratoriums: they simply delayed the removal process in situations where tenants failed to pay rent (46). Rent payments would still become due, and landlords were often permitted to file evictions, even if they could not carry them out immediately, which would give notice to the renters. (40, 46). These programs, nevertheless, staved off what could have been a tidal wave of homelessness in the wake of COVID-19 (47).

Statutory changes by State during COVID-19

During the COVID-19 pandemic, states took heightened notice of the importance of housing. The federal funds targeted to addressing housing stability were unprecedented, and states were required to employ these resources to keep individuals and families housed (48). Nearly every state channeled those federal funds to rent assistance, with all states adopting some form of eviction moratorium, such as the CARES Act or CDC moratoriums, or implementing an state-specific process of tenant protection (which was permitted if the state's provisions provided more protection for the tenant than the CDC moratorium) (40). A handful of states took more substantial steps to prevent evictions than outlined in the CARES Act or CDC moratoriums, enacting laws that could impact systemic issues that have historically facilitated avoidable evictions.

Maine, for example, enacted a program by statute in October 2021called "An Act to Prevent Homelessness by Establishing an Eviction Mediation Program" (49). This program gives tenants the right to alternative dispute resolution (ADR) (49). ADR is a way for parties to come to terms outside of trial, without the involvement of the court. Oftentimes, if ADR is successful, parties can agree to terms that a court could not grant, such as a payment plan, or extra time to move out. Additionally, the law outlines specifically what the notice must contain; this includes a statement within the notice highlighting that either party may request mediation through a court-approved mediation request form (49).

Additionally, the form must include clear language describing the eviction process that must be followed, a statement that failure to appear at any scheduled court date may result in judgment for the landlord (i.e., eviction), a list of rental assistance programs to residential tenants, and resources that provide housing counseling (49).

Maine's amendments are significant, when contrasted to landlord-tenant laws in Georgia – a southeastern state with limited protection of tenants' rights. For example, similar notices in Georgia include only the date the notice is served, the landlord's name, the tenants name and address, the reason for the notice, verification that the landlord demanded possession of the property and was refused, and the total amount of rent and other charges due (50). In

Georgia, tenants are left with information they likely already know, and many questions about what their rights are and what they can do to rectify the issue. The more detailed nature of Maine's notice gives tenants information they need to make decisions about their homes, and how to move forward in ways that may protect their access to safe and affordable housing.

The right to ADR or mediation can be outcome-determinative to an eviction action, meaning that these agreements can result in a remedy without the court being involved in any proceedings whatsoever. These procedures allow a full exploration of options, resulting in an outcome favorable to both parties. This holds especially true for tenants, who are generally inexperienced in navigating the court system. Thus, a notice to tenants that provides mediation information promises a forum in which tenants are provided an opportunity to fully share their concerns and circumstances. For Max, mediation would give her and her landlord the ability to share their goals, what they want, and to share in the context of a conversation so she and her landlord can make decisions about how best to proceed. If Max lived in Maine and fell behind on rent, she and her landlord would be able to, with the help of a mediator, agree to more favorable terms. These terms could include extra time to move out, or some charges on her account reduced.

Default judgment is when a court rules in favor of a plaintiff (property owner or landlord) if a defendant (tenant) fails to respond to a court summons or does not appear in court (24). To minimize default judgements from occurring, Arizona enacted a law that gives tenants the right to appear virtually (51). In the housing context specifically, virtual appearances make it easier for individuals to attend hearings, making it theoretically more likely for tenants to appear at hearings and avoid default judgment. Many people who struggle with housing also work low-wage jobs that are inflexible regarding time off yet have several personal responsibilities to attend throughout the day. Getting "leave time" to attend court can be difficult, and potentially embarrassing (52). In order to attend court, individuals may forego wages at work, pay someone to take care of their children, or may not have access to transportation (53, 54). The ability to attend court online gives people easier access to the courtroom where their case can be decided on facts, instead of an automatic dismissal of the case for failure to attend the court hearing (55). Forcing Max to attend hearings in person, creates another impediment to keeping her in her home.

Connecticut now has "an act concerning the right to counsel in eviction proceedings" giving tenants facing eviction a right to an attorney's assistance throughout eviction proceedings (56). The court system is confusing; providing legal counsel to assist in navigating the eviction process can be more helpful than relying on self-study (9). In Connecticut, tenants receive a copy of a brochure approved by the state judicial department discussing the legal representation available to them at the time of receiving notice (57). Eligible tenants (those who are indigent and who occupy a dwelling unit by right or privilege and exclude the owner of the dwelling unit) at risk of eviction have access to legal representation at no cost (57).

Washington state also enacted a law in April 2021 that provides legal representation for indigent tenants in eviction cases (58). Another new Washington law limits the reasons for an eviction (59). Often, tenants are not aware of the counterclaims or defenses they may assert to defend themselves against an eviction notice. Attorneys can help tenants like Max know their rights, navigate the legal system, and raise applicable claims and appropriate defenses.

In Georgia, by contrast, there is no right to a court-appointed attorney in civil proceedings such as evictions. Without access to a pro bono (gratuitous) legal services lawyer, tenants are left to their own knowledge of the eviction process, making them increasingly reliant on internet research and social media (when available) for legal problems, the reliance on which may be questionable (60). Such methods of research can be faulty because landlord tenant law is dictated by the states; tenants inexperienced in legal research may mistakenly believe that rights existing in one state must also exist in their own.

Maryland has enacted a law giving residential tenants the right to an attorney (much like Washington and Connecticut) (61). Under the Maryland Code, covered individuals will have access to legal representation for proceedings to evict or terminate tenancy (62). The law provides legal representation for appeals as well, and designates that representation begin as soon as possible after notice, at initiation of an eviction proceeding, or when a designated organization determines proceedings related to constructive eviction (i.e., when a property is deemed uninhabitable) can occur (62). For example, if the inside of a home is so covered in mold, though a writ of possession has not been issued by the landlord, a person cannot reasonably be expected to stay and they are, as a result, “constructively evicted.” In contrast, proving constructive eviction in the state of Georgia requires: 1) proof that the landlord’s failure to keep the unit repaired has resulted in the unit becoming unfit for a tenant to live; 2) the unit cannot be restored to a fit condition by ordinary repairs and 3) the tenant has moved out of the premises as a result (63, 64). Warranties of habitability are guarantees that the property is livable and without need of major repairs. Most states have one, and Maryland’s includes provisions that the landlord ensure sewage disposal facilities and must eliminate rodent infestations occurring in two or more units. In Georgia, though technically a warranty of habitability exists, it is lacking, making constructive eviction a hard defense to prove (65).

The organization that oversees the legal representation also "shall develop" a pamphlet in English and other languages describing the legal rights of tenants and the access to counsel established under the Maryland Code (66). It provides additional information on resources available to tenants (66). The tenant must receive this required pamphlet simultaneous with notice of the landlord's eviction action (66).

Among New Jersey renters, expiration of the Statewide moratorium on evictions resulted in as many as 300,000 renters being subject to an eviction proceeding, disproportionately impacting Black and Latino residents of New Jersey (67). As a result, the legislature found that the "provision of free legal services would be one of the most effective ways to address the ongoing eviction crisis" (67). Thus, New Jersey likewise implemented a law giving tenants right to counsel, with Legislative appropriation of monies to law schools in New Jersey (Seton Hall and Rutgers). These monies serve to establish experiential housing advocacy programs that provide free legal services to tenants in need of housing assistance (67, 68). Though not required to do so, both schools used funds to implement Housing Advocacy Clinics under the "Housing Justice Project" (69).

Another legislative change New Jersey enacted, a form of record sealing, has since fallen away, but provided a major relief for tenants during the height of the pandemic (70). Sealing is when a judge makes a record no longer publicly available (24). In New Jersey from March 1, 2020, through August 31, 2021, landlords were not allowed to report delayed rent to crediting agencies, they could not sell the debt, and they could not disclose non-payment of rent to others. At the time of this paper, New Jersey is considering adopting legislation that would seal landlord-tenant proceedings until judgment is entered, though it could stay sealed even after judgment should the tenant prove a breach of warranty of habitability or that the complaint from the landlord was unlawful (71). Ensuring evictions proceedings are kept confidential except for the final judgment – should the tenant be evicted – provides an equitable way forward for the tenant, while still keeping important information available to future landlords.

Additionally, prospective landlords in New Jersey were not allowed to deny renting to a person who was unable to pay rent during the covered period. By using federal funds for rent assistance, landlords were not forced into bankruptcy, or other economic crises (70). This measure also helped landlords who, lacking steady income from tenants facing economic hardship, saw their own share of financial struggles throughout the pandemic.

Nevada also enacted a law requiring record sealing for evictions and other adverse actions during the COVID-19 pandemic, permitting tenants to assert affirmative defenses relating to their rental assistance (72). These affirmative defenses have the effect of mandating a judge to keep an eviction from moving forward. Under Nevada law, if a court granted an action for summary eviction during the COVID-19 emergency, the court would seal the eviction case court file (72). Moreover, the statute allowed the record to be sealed automatically, meaning the tenant did not have to affirmatively act to have their record sealed (72). This law lapsed on May 20, 2022, at the end of the COVID-19 emergency (72). Had Max lived in Nevada when she got COVID, even if she was evicted due to lack of payment because of contracting COVID, she could have submitted an affirmative defense (citing her COVID diagnosis and subsequent need to isolate at home for two weeks without pay) to have her record sealed. Once she was back at work, she would be able to apply for new housing, without fear of her children living without a roof over their heads, or of a new landlord learning of her eviction.

New York law provides a "sufficient number of pro se clerks of the housing part (or department) to assist persons without counsel" (73). People who lack legal representation have clerks who can assist them filing court papers, provide information on court procedure, and advise individuals to seek administrative relief, though these clerks may provide other assistance as well (73). Litigants also receive information and notices, available in several languages, giving tenants a better chance at understanding the information that they are receiving (73). For someone like Max, having clerks who can provide information, file papers, and give guidance as to court processes can go a long way in assisting Max as she navigates the process of responding to an eviction notice.

Hypothesis

Evictions have a detrimental impact on subsequent housing and childhood mental health outcomes, by creating and compounding various Adverse Childhood Experiences including the cycle of poverty (ACEs). Therefore, states implementing tenant protection laws can help decrease ACEs and childhood mental illness.

Our study

Evaluating the laws implemented by the various states required showing a relationship between tenant protection laws and children's mental illness. This project sought to measure five tenant protection laws enacted across eight states, and how these statutory changes may have improved children's mental health, by 1) investigating the connection between tenant protection laws and child poverty, 2) examining the literature that establishes the connection between poverty and children's mental health and 3) utilizing two regression models. One regression model measured these five tenant protection laws and childhood poverty rates, by state, between 2019 and 2021. The second regression model measured the five tenant protection laws and the change in rates of households (with children) where there was little or no confidence in ability to pay next rent or mortgage payment on-time, by state, between 2020 and 2022. Rates of 1) childhood poverty and 2) households with children where there was little or no confidence in ability to pay their next rent or mortgage payment on-time were obtained from the Annie E Casey Foundation's Kids Count Data Center.

Findings

Figure 2 assesses changes in poverty from 2019 to 2020, showing a point before the tenant protection laws were in place, and a point in time after. Few changes occurred in the two-year span, and the results showed no statistically significant correlation between the tenant protection laws and poverty rate.

Regression analysis of Tenant Protection Laws and changes in poverty rate (2019-2021)

- X-Variable (slope): -0.75 (-1.65, 0.15), $p = 0.10$
- Results showed no statistically significant correlation between tenant protection laws and poverty rates in these eight states. The second regression analysis measured the change in households with children where there was little or no confidence in ability to pay their next rent or mortgage on time. Results showed no statistically significant correlation between tenant protection and households with children where there was little or no confidence in ability to pay their next rent or mortgage payment on time in these eight states.

A downward trend in households with children, where there was little or no confidence in ability to pay their next rent or mortgage payment, was demonstrated over time (after enacting tenant protection laws across the aforementioned eight states).

Regression analysis of Tenant Protection Laws and change in rates of households with children where there was little or no confidence in ability to pay their next rent or mortgage payment on time (2020-2022)

- X-Variable (slope): -0.02 (-0.64, 0.022), $p = 0.325$
- Results showed no statistically significant correlation between tenant protection laws and households with children where there was little or no confidence in ability to pay their next rent or mortgage payment on time in these eight states.

Conclusion

Analysis of tenant protection laws implemented in eight states in 2021 (in response to COVID-19 pandemic) did not significantly correlate to changes in poverty rates between 2019-2021 or changes in tenant confidence on ability to pay their next rent or mortgage payment between 2020-2022 respectively. However, effects on poverty and ability to pay rent or mortgage are not single-factor issues, and measuring the impacts of a single law on systemic and complicated issues will not give the full picture. Such outcomes involve various other existing confounders, such as job and wage loss occurring during the pandemic, transition from a two-parent to a single parent home, having a child, or a family member developing disabilities. Moreover, as of this publication, these laws have only been in place for two years at most; thus, their residual impact remains to be seen in coming years. Finally, some laws are COVID-specific, meaning they will not have as much impact as public and statutory responses to the pandemic fade. Further, this study had a low representation model, with only eight out of 50 states serving as the dependent variable (74).

Suggestions for future

To gain better perspective on what anti-eviction or tenant protection laws can impact, including more variables in the regression analysis could lead to more specific findings. Variables might include factors such as whether the family status was impacted by COVID or not, whether anyone in the household developed a chronic health issue, whether the home is or became multigenerational, or whether a tenant faced a disability. A cross sectional study comparing one state enacting tenant protection laws to another that has not enacted such laws could better highlight differences in poverty changes over time. Other options include looking at localities, considering local-level policies that have been implemented, and conducting interviews with landlord-tenant lawyers in each of the jurisdictions to ascertain whether they perceive that the newly enacted tenant protections have provided tenants with greater protections and, as a result, helped prevent the eviction of families.

The law can be a powerful tool in bringing about social change. Statutory changes to the law can help address housing insecurity, even if it cannot fix the entire system of poverty and homelessness. The laws discussed show a shift in policy and are perhaps indicative of changes society favor. Max, and other women like her, are, in most states, left to a legal system that gives tenants few rights when falling upon hard times. The goal of this review is to encourage other states to consider policy and statutory changes that consider the children caught in the mix of evictions and help keep them out of harm's way—the harm that often results in part from substandard housing.

Acknowledgements

Disclosure statements: the authors have no financial relationships relevant to this article to disclose. The authors have no conflicts of interest to disclose. The preparation for this project and manuscript review was supported by the Break the Cycle of Health Disparities Program of the Southeast PEHSU at Emory University and Break the Cycle of Health Disparities, Inc. Use of names, trade names, or other persons is for identification and citation purposes only and does not imply endorsement by this paper, Break the Cycle, Georgia State University College of Law, or Emory University.

References

[1] Evictions. Fulton County Georgia. URL: ttps://www.fultoncountyga.gov/inside-fulton-county/fulton-county-departments/marshal/evictions.

[2] O'Connell A. Consequences of illegal evictions. NOLO. URL: https://www.nolo.com/legal-encyclopedia/consequences-of-illegal-evictions.html.

[3] Balch O. Landlords are powerful. Here's a way renters are regaining some control. HuffPost 2018. URL: https://www.huffpost.com/entry/rate-your-landlord-power-tenants-rentals_n_5be06c7be4b09d43e321620c.

[4] Centers for Disease Control and Prevention. Preventing adverse childhood experiences (ACEs): Leveraging the best available evidence 2019. URL: https://www.cdc.gov/violenceprevention/pdf/preventingACES.pdf.

[5] Schupmann W. How housing quality affects child mental health. Housing Matters 2017. URL: https://housingmatters.urban.org/articles/how-housing-quality-affects-child-mental-health.

[6] The Eviction Lab. URL: https://evictionlab.org.

[7] Gromis A. Eviction: Intersection of poverty, inequality, and housing. URL: https://www.un.org/development/desa/dspd/wp-content/uploads/sites/22/2019/05/GROMIS_Ashley_Paper.pdf.

[8] National Law Center on Homelessness and Poverty. Protect tenants, prevent homelessness. URL: https://homelesslaw.org/wp-content/uploads/2018/10/ProtectTenants2018.pdf.

[9] Eviction Defense Collaborative. Our work through the stories of our community. URL: https://evictiondefense.org/about/impact/.

[10] Rocket Lawyer. Free Georgia eviction notice template: Sample and FAQs. URL: https://www.rocketlawyer.com/real-estate/landlords/eviction/document/eviction-notice/ga.

[11] Stewart, M. How rent withholding works. NOLO. URL: https://www.nolo.com/legal-encyclopedia/how-rent-withholding-works.html.

[12] Leifheit KM. JAMA Network 2023. URL: https://jamanetwork.com/journals/jamanetworkopen/fullarticle/2803676.

[13] Hepburn P, Louis R, Desmond M. Racial and gender disparities among evicted Americans. Eviction Lab 2020. URL: https://evictionlab.org/demographics-of-eviction/;

[14] Benfer EA. US eviction policy is harming children: The case for sustainable eviction prevention to promote health equity. Bill of Health 2022. URL: https://blog.petrieflom.law.harvard.edu/2022/11/02/pandemic-eviction-policy-children.

[15] Lundberg I, Donnelly L. How many children experience eviction during childhood? Housing Matters 2019. URL: https://housingmatters.urban.org/research-summary/how-many-children-experience-eviction-during-childhood.

[16] Nellis A. Mass incarceration trends. The Sentencing Project 2023. URL: https://www.sentencingproject.org/reports/mass-incarceration-trends;

[17] Solomon M, Baldassari E. Why Black women are more likely to face eviction. KQED 2022. URL: https://www.kqed.org/news/11905386/why-black-women-are-more-likely-to-face-eviction.

[18] Desmond M. Evicted: Poverty and profit in the American City. London: Penguin Books, 2016.

[19] Why eviction matters. Eviction Lab. URL: https://evictionlab.org/why-eviction-matters.

[20] Benfer EA, Koehler R, Mark A, Nazzaro V, Alexander AK, Hepburn P, et al. Assessing state eviction prevention policies in response to COVID-19. Eviction Lab 2022. URL: https://evictionlab.org/assessing-state-eviction-prevention-covid-19/.

[21] Hinshaw TE. Georgia Jurisprudence. Thompson Reuters. Eagan, MN: Lawyers Cooperative Publishing, 2014-2023.

[22] Mott R. Evictions increase in Katrina's wake. NBC News 2005. URL: https://www.nbcnews.com/id/wbna9889318.

[23] Benfer EA, Vlahov D, Long MY, Walker-Wells E, Pottenger JL, Gonsalves G, et al. Eviction, health inequity, and the spread of COVID-19: Housing policy as a primary pandemic mitigation strategy. J Urban Health 2021;98(1):1-12.

[24] Garner BA ed. Black's law dictionary. Eagan, MN: Thomson Reuters business, 2019.

[25] Peiffer E. Why we need to stop evictions before they happen. Housing Matters 2018. URL: https://housingmatters.urban.org/feature/why-we-need-stop-evictions-they-happen.

[26] Code of conduct for United States judges. United States Courts 2019. URL: https://www.uscourts.gov/sites/default/files/code_of_conduct_for_united_states_judges_effective_march_12_2019.pdf.

[27] Desmond M, Gershenson C, Kiviat B. Forced relocation and residential instability among urban renters. Soc Serv Rev 2015;89(2):227-62.

[28] Landlord-Tenant Law. Legal Information Institute. URL: https://www.law.cornell.edu/wex/landlord-tenant_law.

[29] Militello A. How to look up evictions (and prevent disastrous rentals!). RentPrep 2023. URL: https://rentprep.com/blog/evictions/how-to-look-up-evictions/.

[30] So W. Which information matters? Measuring landlord assessment of tenant screening reports. Hous Policy Debate 2022;33(6):1-27.

[31] White J. How long does an eviction stay on your credit report? Experian 2023. URL: https://www.experian.com/blogs/ask-experian/how-long-does-eviction-stay-on-report.

[32] How long can information, like eviction actions and lawsuits, stay on my tenant screening record? Consumer Financial Protection Bureau 2021. URL: https://www.consumerfinance.gov/ask-cfpb/how-long-can-information-like-eviction-actions-and-lawsuits-stay-on-my-tenant-screening-record-en-2104/.

[33] For what cause may a landlord evict a tenant? Legal Services Corporation Eviction Laws Database. URL: https://www.lsc.gov/initiatives/effect-state-local-laws-evictions/lsc-eviction-laws-database.

[34] Mateyka P, Yoo, J. Share of income needed to pay rent increased the most for low-income households from 2019 to 2021. United States Census Bureau 2023. URL: https://www.census.gov/library/stories/2023/03/low-income-renters-spent-larger-share-of-income-on-rent.html.

[35] Alcantara C. Rent is rising. See how much prices are up in your area. Washington Post 2022. URL: https://www.washingtonpost.com/business/interactive/2022/rising-rent-prices.

[36] Gates L. Child homelessness: A growing crisis. Substance Abuse and Mental Health Services Administration 2016. URL: https://www.samhsa.gov/homelessness-programs-resources/hpr-resources/child-homelessness-growing-crisis;

[37] Vásquez-Vera H, Palència L, Magna I, Mena C, Neira J, Borrell C. The threat of home eviction and its effects on health through the equity lens: A systematic review. Soc Sci Med 2017;175:199-208.

[38] Acharya B, Bhatta D, Dhakal C. The risk of eviction and the mental health outcomes among the US adults. Prev Med Rep 2022;29:101981.

[39] Preventing adverse childhood experiences. Center for Disease Control 2020. URL: https://www.cdc.gov/violenceprevention/aces/fastfact.html.

[40] Federal Eviction Moratoriums in Response to the COVID-19 Pandemic. Congressional Research Service 2021. URL: https://crsreports.congress.gov/product/pdf/IN/IN11516;

[41] CARES Act: Temporary Moratorium on Eviction Filings 2020 15 U.S.C.A. § 9058.

[42] The CDC eviction moratorium has ended: Learn your options. Consumer Financial Protection Bureau 2021. URL: https://www.consumerfinance.gov/about-us/blog/the-cdc-eviction-moratorium-has-ended-learn-your-options/.

[43] Emergency Rental Assistance Program. US Department of the Treasury. URL: https://home.treasury.gov/policy-issues/coronavirus/assistance-for-state-local-and-tribal-governments/emergency-rental-assistance-program.

[44] Hepburn P, Jin O, Fish J, Lemmerman E, Alexander AK, Desmond M. Preliminary analysis: Eviction filing patterns in 2021. Eviction Lab 2022. URL: https://evictionlab.org/us-eviction-filing-patterns-2021

[45] Hepburn P, Haas J, Graetz N, Louis R, Rutan DQ, Alexander AK, et al. COVID-era policies cut eviction filings by more than half. Eviction Lab 2023. URL: https://evictionlab.org/covid-era-policies-cut-eviction-filings-by-more-than-half.

[46] Cunningham MK, Greene S. The CDC took an important step to halt evictions because of COVID-19. But that's only half the battle. Urban Institute 2020. URL: https://www.urban.org/urban-wire/cdc-took-important-step-halt-evictions-because-covid-19-thats-only-half-battle.

[47] Capps K. Housing instability spiked during the pandemic. Homelessness didn't. Bloomberg 2023. URL: https://www.bloomberg.com/news/articles/2023-08-22/how-covid-era-housing-relief-prevented-an-eviction-wave.

[48] Pandemic relief: The emergency rental assistance program. Congressional Research Service. URL: https://crsreports.congress.gov/product/pdf/R/R46688.

[49] Commencement of Action 2023 (Me. Rev. Stat. 14 § 6004).

[50] What should I know about evictions? Georgia Leal Aid. URL: https://www.georgialegalaid.org/resource/what-to-know-about-evictions#2.

[51] Residential Eviction Information Sheet 2023 (17B A.R.S. Rules Proc. Evic. Act., App. A)

[52] Desmond M, Gershenson C. Housing and employment insecurity among the working poor. Harvard University 2016. URL: https://scholar.harvard.edu/files/mdesmond/files/desmondgershenson.sp2016.pdf?m=1452638824.
[53] Holder S. At Philadelphia Eviction Court, showing up on time is half the battle. Bloomberg 2022. URL: https://www.bloomberg.com/news/articles/2022-07-22/why-poor-public-transit-can-bring-more-evictions;
[54] Levin M. Tenants with long commutes to court more likely to be evicted, study finds. Marketplace 2022. URL: https://www.marketplace.org/2022/06/10/tenants-with-long-commutes-to-court-more-likely-to-be-evicted-study-finds/.
[55] Bannon A, Adelstein J. The impact of video proceedings on fairness and access to justice in court. Brennan Center for Justice 2020. URL: https://www.brennancenter.org/our-work/research-reports/impact-video-proceedings-fairness-and-access-justice-court.
[56] An act concerning the right to counsel in eviction proceedings, the validity of inland wetlands permits in relation to certain other land use approvals, and extending the time of expiration of certain land use permits 2021. URL:
[57] https://www.cga.ct.gov/2021/ACT/PA/PDF/2021PA-00034-R00HB-06531-PA.PDF
[58] An Act Concerning the Right to Counsel in Eviction Proceedings 2021. https://www.cga.ct.gov/2021/TOB/H/PDF/2021HB-06531-R00-HB.PDF.
[59] RCW 59.18.640: Indigent tenants. URL: https://app.leg.wa.gov/RCW/default.aspx?cite=59.18.640.
[60] RCW 59.18.650: Eviction of tenant, refusal to continue tenancy, end of periodic tenancy—Cause—Notice—Penalties. URL: https://app.leg.wa.gov/RCW/default.aspx?cite=59.18.650.
[61] Justice Needs and Satisfaction in the United States of America 2021 Legal problems in daily life. The Hague Institution for Innovation of Law 2021. URL: https://iaals.du.edu/sites/default/files/documents/publications/justice-needs-and-satisfaction-us.pdf.
[62] Access to legal representation 2021 (MD Code, Real Property, § 8-902).
[63] Provision of access to legal representation 2021 (MD Code, Real Property, § 8-904).
[64] Jenkins v. Brice (1998)
[65] Georgia Landlord-Tenant Handbook. A landlord-tenant guide to the State's rental laws revised. State of Georgia 2021. URL: https://www.dca.ga.gov/sites/default/files/2-15-21_handbook_final_draft.pdf.
[66] Miller A. Georgia bill would protect tenants facing unhealthy living conditions. WABE 2019. URL: https://www.wabe.org/ga-bill-would-protect-tenants-facing-unhealthy-living-conditions;
[67] Informational pamphlet 2021 (MD Code, Real Property, § 8-905).
[68] Legislative findings and declarations relating to experiential housing advocacy programs 2021 (N.J.S.A. 22A:2-51a).
[69] Experiential housing advocacy programs; services provided; implementation and supervision; application; report 2021 (N.J.S.A. 22A:2-51b).

[70] Housing Justice Project Releases Report on Landlord-Tenant Reform in New Jersey. Rutgers Law 2022. Available from: https://law.rutgers.edu/news/housing-justice-project-releases-report-landlord-tenant-reform-new-jersey.
[71] Governor Murphy signs sweeping housing eviction prevention and utility assistance bill. State of New Jersey 2021. URL: https://www.nj.gov/governor/news/news/562021/20210804b.shtml.
[72] An act concerning the confidentiality of landlord-tenant court records and supplementing Title 2A of the New Jersey Statutes. New Jersey Legislature 2022. URL: https://pub.njleg.gov/Bills/2022/S0500/392_I1.HTM.
[73] Unlawful detainer: Sealing of eviction case court file under certain circumstances; notice to surrender must not be made available for public inspection 2021 (N.R.S. 40.2545).
[74] Housing Part 2022 (McKinney's NY City Civ. Ct. Act § 110).
[75] Mckernan SM, Ratcliffe C, Cellini S. Transitioning in and out of poverty. The Urban Institute 2009. URL: https://www.urban.org/sites/default/files/publication/30636/411956-Transitioning-In-and-Out-of-Poverty.PDF.
[76] Trusted well-being data on children and young people in The United States. Annie E Casey Foundation Kids Count Data Center. URL: https://datacenter.aecf.org.

Chapter 4

Neighborhood child opportunity, air pollution and telomere length among children

Austin Le, MS[1]
Stephanie Holm, MD, PhD, MPH[2]
Morgan Ye, MPH[3]
Nicole R Bush, PhD[4,5]
Danielle Hessler, PhD[6]
Kadiatou Koita, MD, MS[7]
Monica Bucci, MD[7]
Dayna Long, MD[5,8]
Neeta Thakur, MD, MPH[3]
and Rosemarie de la Rosa, PhD, MPH[1,3,*]

[1]Environmental Health Sciences Division, School of Public Health, University of California, Berkeley, California, United States of America
[2]Western States Pediatric Environmental Health Specialty Unit, San Francisco, California, United States of America
[3]Division of Pulmonary and Critical Care Medicine, Department of Medicine, University of California, San Francisco, California, United States of America
[4]Department of Psychiatry and Behavioral Science, University of California, San Francisco, California, United States of America
[5]Department of Pediatrics, University of California, San Francisco, California, United States of America
[6]Department of Family and Community Medicine, University of California, San Francisco, California, United States of America
[7]Center for Youth Wellness, San Francisco, California, United States of America
[8]UCSF Benioff Children's Hospital Oakland, San Francisco, California, United States of America

[*] Corresponding Author's E-mail: rmd1025@berkeley.edu

In: Neighborhoods: Impact on Child Health and Development
Editors: I Leslie Rubin and Joav Merrick
ISBN: 979-8-89530-834-9

Neighborhood resources are associated with positive health outcomes among children. Telomere length (TL) serves as a marker of stress-related, biological aging and inversely associated with adverse environmental factors. We set out to examine the association between neighborhood child opportunity and residential ambient air pollution with TL among children and assess whether this association is modified by neighborhood child opportunity. We studies children (1-11 years of age) from the Pediatric Adverse Childhood Experiences (ACEs) and Resiliency Study cohort. Methods: Neighborhood Child Opportunity Index (COI) and ambient particulate matter ($PM_{2.5}$) concentrations were matched to residential locations for the twelve months prior to biospecimen collection. Relative buccal TL was measured using quantitative polymerase chain reaction. Multivariable linear regression models were used to examine for associations between neighborhood COI (continuous and categorical) and TL adjusting for sociodemographics. The study sample consisted of 299 children (45.8% girls, mean age of 6.0 years [standard deviation: 3.4]) with median COI of 28.0 [IQR: 41.5], median 12-month prior $PM_{2.5}$ concentrations of 11.8 $\mu g/m^3$ [IQR: 2.5], and median TL of 0.1 [IQR: 0.03]. Continuous and categorical COI and COI domains were not associated with TL. Average 12-month prior residential $PM_{2.5}$ was associated with shorter TL ($ß$ = -0.02, 95% CI: -0.04, -0.01). The interaction between COI and $PM_{2.5}$ exposure on TL was nonsignificant ($p = 0.82$). Neighborhood resources were not found to have an impact on physiologic aging among young children. Future longitudinal studies are warranted to explore the long-term impact of neighborhood environments on health outcomes as children advance into adolescence and adulthood.

Introduction

Neighborhood opportunities, such as proximal access to healthcare, greenspace, and early childhood development centers, are conducive to creating healthy environments for children to grow, develop and thrive. The Child Opportunity Index (COI) was developed as a nationwide scoring tool to quantify these assets by geographic area (1) and allows a snapshot of the resources available in a child's neighborhood that may impact their health and development. Greater neighborhood opportunity, measured using the COI, has been associated with multiple positive health outcomes for neighborhoods, such as lower asthma hospitalization rates (2) and lower adolescent metabolic risk (3). How neighborhood opportunity operates on health and whether the mechanism for this benefit occurs at the cellular level is not known.

Telomeres are nucleotide-protein caps at the ends of chromosomes that shorten with each round of cellular division, and telomere length (TL) is a well-known biomarker of physiologic aging (4). TL inherently shortens across the lifespan, and shorter TL has been associated with age-related diseases (e.g., cardiovascular disease and Alzheimer's disease) and mortality (5). In contrast, longer TL has been associated with greater risk for major types of cancer (6, 7). In the first two years of life, children experience the greatest telomere shortening during this period of rapid growth (8). Thus, early life may be a critical window for identifying both risk factors and interventions that may contribute to TL trajectories across the lifespan.

There is growing evidence of the impact of adverse neighborhood characteristics on TL (9). Objective measures of area-level neighborhood disadvantage, such as less walkability (10), neighborhood deprivation (11-13), and residential crowding, stability, and mobility (14) have all been associated with shorter TL among adults. Subjective measures, such as perceived neighborhood problems (15), perceived poor neighborhood quality (16, 17), and perceived poor neighborhood social environment (18) have also been associated with shorter TL among adults. Long-term accumulation of perceived neighborhood stressors has been associated with shorter TL among female adults in West Scotland (19).

Studies examining relationships between neighborhood factors and TL among children are limited, though they do agree with the findings of those conducted among adults. Additionally, most studies in children using area-level indices are deprivation/disadvantage-based (9). For instance, caregiver-reported perceived neighborhood disorder has been reported to be associated with shorter TL among children ages 4-14 years (20). Furthermore, within 500 meters of children's (ages 5-16 years) homes, the density of liquor/convenience stores and rates of violent crime and domestic violence were reported to be negatively associated with TL (21). One such neighborhood asset (proximity and duration of exposure to greenspace) has been observed to be associated with longer TL among preschool children (22). Given the dearth of studies that examine the comprehensive impact of positive neighborhood-level factors on TL among children, further research is warranted to characterize this relationship.

Currently, there is a scarcity of research examining neighborhood assets or resources that buffer TL attrition. A prior longitudinal study found that improvements in neighborhood-level socioeconomic status was associated with a slower TL attrition over 10 years (23). Therefore, greater neighborhood child opportunity may be associated with reduced TL attrition.

Harmful environmental exposures are highly prevalent in communities that have been historically marginalized and disadvantaged (24, 25). Children living in suboptimal, disinvested neighborhood environments— a result of structural racism— are more likely to be exposed to harmful toxicants (26, 27) and may be caught in a cycle of continued exposure for themselves and for succeeding generations (28). Our group has previously demonstrated that annual exposure to fine particulate matter ($PM_{2.5}$) is associated with shorter TL among children ages 1-11 years (29), which agrees with findings from prior studies (30-33). As a way to "break the cycle" of the disparities in air pollution exposure, neighborhood disadvantage, and biological aging, we postulate that residing in neighborhoods with greater resources (educational, social and economic, and health and environment-related) may buffer against the adverse effect of $PM_{2.5}$ on TL (see figure 1).

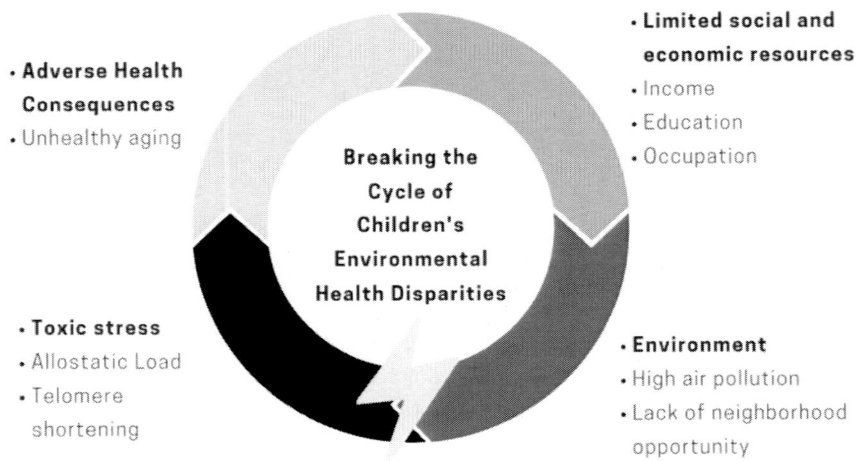

Figure 1. Concept map of "Breaking the Cycle" of environmental health disparities among children. This study examines relationships between neighborhood child opportunity and air pollution with telomere length, a physiological biomarker of aging. We posit that greater opportunities could buffer the adverse.

We hypothesize that exposure to greater neighborhood opportunity is associated with greater TL and that exposure to greater neighborhood opportunity buffers telomere shortening associated with living in environments with high ambient air pollution exposure. Here, we examine the independent effect of neighborhood opportunity on TL among children enrolled in the Pediatric ACEs Screening and Resiliency Study (PEARLS)

(34). PEARLS is a longitudinal cohort study that predominantly consisted of non-Hispanic Black children and their families recruited during well-child care at the University of California, San Francisco (UCSF) Benioff Children's Hospital Oakland Primary Care Clinic. Detailed information about the study can be found elsewhere (34). In this study, we also explored whether the adverse association between $PM_{2.5}$ and TL was modified by the amount of objective neighborhood opportunity.

Our study

The present observational, cross-sectional study involves participants from PEARLS. Between March 2017 and October 2018, a total of 555 children aged three months to 11 years, along with their caregivers, were enrolled into PEARLS. Enrolled participants were randomly allocated into adversity screening or control arms. Biospecimen collection took place in both groups during a separate study visit scheduled within one month of initial enrollment, with buccal swabs collected from participants at the one-month follow-up (n = 399). Children under the age of one year were excluded from the analysis as they had less than 12 months of postnatal air pollution exposure data available (n = 32). The analysis was further limited to participants who had geocoded addresses available and DNA specimens that met the quality control criteria outlined below (n = 307), and to participants with available air pollution exposure estimates, to reach the final analytical sample (n = 299). Caregivers provided informed, written consent to participate in the study. The study was approved by the UCSF Benioff Oakland institutional review board (IRB), with UC Berkeley serving as a relying institution (#3941). The protocol number for the Pediatric ACEs and Resiliency Study is 21-33697.

Neighborhood child opportunity

The Child Opportunity Index (COI) was used to measure the level of neighborhood opportunity in each participant's residential census tract. The COI is a multidimensional scoring tool comprising 29 indicators relevant to children's health and development (1). These indicators were grouped into three domains of census-tract level opportunity: 1) Education opportunity, which includes number of early childhood education centers, school poverty, and third grade reading proficiency, etc.; 2) Health and environment opportunity, which includes access to green space, ambient average microparticle and ozone concentration, access to health food, etc.; and 3) Social and economic opportunity, which includes public assistance rate, median household income, employment rate, etc. Each indicator was standardized and weighted by how strongly it predicted census-tract level economic and health outcomes. These weighted scores were then summed to create domain-specific and overall scores for each census tract. The overall and domain COI scores were modeled as both continuous variables and categorically using California state-normed quintiles ("Very low", "Low", "Moderate", "High", "Very high"). In the present analysis, adjacent categories (e.g., "Very low" and "Low" or "Very high" and "High") with <10% of the analytical sample size were combined.

Ambient residential air pollution

Fine particulate matter concentrations were assigned to participant residential addresses provided by caregivers at study baseline. Monthly ground-level $PM_{2.5}$ estimates were derived from publicly available datasets provided by the Atmospheric Composition Group at Washington University in St Louis that used a combination of remotely sensed data from satellites, chemical transport models, and ground-based measurements in a geographically weighted regression model at roughly one km resolution (35). For the 12 months prior to biospecimen collection, a time-weighted average of $PM_{2.5}$ exposure using data from each residential address was estimated using the following equation:

$$Average\ PM_{2.5}\ exposure = \frac{\sum_{i=1}^{n}(residential\ PM_{2.5})_i * \frac{\#\ of\ days\ exposed_i}{total\ \#\ of\ days_i}}{\sum_{i=1}^{n}\frac{\#\ of\ days\ exposed_i}{total\ \#\ of\ days_i}}$$

Where i represents a given month from 0 to 12 for the months prior to biospecimen collection. The calculation incorporates the proportion of days within each month of the exposure period leading up to the biospecimen collection date. The exposure period spans from the previous year's collection date to the current year's collection date. Monthly weights are assigned based on the proportion of days within each month, except for the collection month, which is proportionally weighted based on the days leading up to the collection date. This approach thus adjusts for varying month lengths.

Telomere length

Buccal swabs were collected from participants using the ORAcollect for Pediatrics collection kit (DNA Genotek, Cat# OC-175) and DNA was extracted using DNA Genotech prepIT-L2P reagents according to the manufacturer's protocol. A NanoDrop® spectrophotometer was used to assess the DNA concentration and quality (OD260/280). Buccal DNA that met minimum concentration values (5ng/µL) and had purity 260/280 values between 1.7-2.0 were used to quantify telomere length. Relative buccal telomere length was quantified using the quantitative polymerase chain reaction (qPCR) method with modifications by O'Callaghan et al. 2011 (36-37). Briefly, samples were assayed in triplicate within the same plate using two separate uniplex qPCR reactions for both the telomeric region (T) and a single-copy gene (S, 36B4). Each qPCR plate contained a reference control DNA sample (1301 cell line DNA), a no template negative control, and T or S standard curves (37). Standard curve amplification efficiencies across all plates were ≥90% for both assays. T/S ratios for each sample was calculated using the delta-delta Ct ($2{-}\Delta\Delta Ct$) method (4). Sample T/S ratios were then normalized to the T/S ratio for the reference control DNA included on every PCR plate to obtain relative buccal TL values. As TL did not follow a normal distribution in the study population, it was log-transformed to meet the normality of residuals criteria for regression analyses. The intraclass correlation coefficient (ICC) was 0.88 for 20 participant samples with repeated measures on two separate plates run in triplicate each time.

Covariates

Covariates for the analysis were chosen based on a directed acyclic graph derived from a comprehensive review of previous literature. Sociodemographic factors were obtained through a caregiver questionnaire administered at the beginning of the study. Child age (continuous) was defined as the age in years at the time of study enrollment. Gender was made categorical and recorded as either "boy" or "girl" based on information provided by the caregiver. Child race/ethnicity (categorical) was determined from the caregiver's selection of available racial/ethnic options and further categorized into the following groups: non-Hispanic Black, Hispanic, two or more races, or other. Caregiver education (categorical) was consolidated into the following attainment categories: "≤ High school/GED," "Some college," and "College graduate." The reference group was selected based on the categories with the highest number of participants.

Statistical analysis

To compare the mean relative buccal TL between categorical and continuous variables, bivariate linear regression was employed. The Kruskal-Wallis test was used for bivariate comparison between overall COI and domain categories with TL. Log-transformed TL was used for all stated analyses. Multivariable linear regression was used to assess the independent association between overall COI and each domain (continuous score and categorical) with TL (continuous) adjusting for individual-level covariates such as child age, gender, caregiver education (proxy for family socioeconomic status), and race that may confound neighborhood-level effects. To evaluate the potential effect measure modification on the association between average $PM_{2.5}$ exposure and TL, an interaction term between average annual $PM_{2.5}$ exposure and overall COI or average annual $PM_{2.5}$ exposure and individual COI domain were included in separate models. Statistical significance was determined at a two-sided threshold of $p < 0.05$ for the main results, while a threshold of $p < 0.10$ was used for interaction tests (38). All statistical analyses were performed using RStudio Version 2022.07.2 (39).

Sensitivity analysis

Given that the context of the PEARLS trial was to inform targeted stress interventions among a highly burdened study population, we assessed early-life adversities as a potential confounder in the association between COI and TL. Early-life adversities were measured using the 17-item Pediatric Adverse Childhood Experiences and Related Life Events Screener (34), which was administered to caregivers and assessed cumulative exposure to experiences of abuse, neglect, household challenges, and social determinants of health. In a sub-sample of participants with available early-life adversities data (n = 195), we included this adversity score (continuous) as a covariate in our multivariable regression models. We also utilized Pearson's correlation tests to assess bivariate correlations.

Our findings

The study sample consisted of 299 children between the ages of 1-11 years with an average age of 6.0 years (SD = 3.4), mostly boys (54.2%), and predominantly non-Hispanic Black (54.2%) (see table 1). The caregiver education level consisted of ≤ High school/ GED (39.5%), some college (39.1%), and ≥ College graduate (21.4%). The median TL was 0.1 with IQR of 0.03. In bivariate analysis, child age was significantly inversely associated with TL (ß = -0.02, 95% CI: -0.03, -0.02), where a one-year increment in age was associated with a 0.02 decrement in TL. TL did not differ significantly by participant gender, race, or caregiver education.

Table 1. Study participant characteristics and associations with telomere length (n = 299)

Characteristic	**N (%)**	**ß (95% CI)**
Child age (years), mean (standard deviation)	6.0 (3.4)	**-0.02 (-0.03, -0.02)***
Gender		
Boy (reference)	162 (54.2)	reference
Girl	137 (45.8)	0.02 (-0.03, 0.07)
Race		
Non-Hispanic Black (reference)	162 (54.2)	reference
Hispanic	73 (24.4)	0.01 (-0.05, 0.07)
Two or more races	39 (13.0)	0.01 (-0.07, 0.08)
Other†	25 (8.4)	-0.06 (-0.15, 0.03)
Caregiver education		
≤ High school/ GED (reference)	118 (39.5)	reference
Some college	117 (39.1)	-0.0 (-0.06, 0.05)
≥College graduate	64 (21.4)	0.02 (-0.05, 0.09)

Abbreviations: **CI,** Confidence Interval; **GED**, General Education Development; **IQR,** interquartile range

* denotes statistically significant at $p<0.05$.

† "Other" is an aggregate race category due to low sample size and is composed of Asian, Middle Eastern/North African, non-Hispanic White, American Indian or Alaskan Native, or prefer not to answer.

Bivariate analyses revealed no statistically significant differences in average TL between overall COI categories or domains (see figure 2). Neither overall COI nor COI domains were associated with TL when modeled continuously and categorically (see table 2).

In multivariable analyses, after adjusting for participant age, gender, race, and caregiver education, annual ambient residential $PM_{2.5}$ was inversely associated with TL where a one-unit increment in average annual $PM_{2.5}$

concentration was associated with a 0.02 decrement in TL (ß = -0.02, 95% CI: -0.04, -0.01) (see table 2).

Table 2. Multivariable adjusted associations between exposures and telomere length

Exposure	Median (IQR)	ß (95% CI)
COI		
Continuous	28 (41.5)	-0.0002 (-0.0012, 0.0008)
Categories, n(%)		
Very Low	100 (33.4)	reference
Low	86 (28.8)	0.0130 (-0.0456, 0.0716)
Moderate	53 (17.7)	-0.0072 (-0.0748, 0.060)
High/ Very High	60 (20.1)	-0.0058 (-0.0765, 0.0650)
Education Opportunity		
Continuous	20 (43)	-0.0006 (-0.0015, 0.0002)
Categories, n(%)		
Very Low	150 (50.2)	reference
Low	44 (14.7)	-0.0278 (-0.0955, 0.0400)
Moderate	49 (16.4)	-0.0424 (-0.1090, 0.0242)
High/Very High	56 (18.7)	-0.0452 (-0.1112, 0.0208)
Health and Environment Opportunity		
Continuous	60 (39)	0.0004 (-0.0005, 0.0014)
Categories, n(%)		
Very Low/ Low	83 (27.8)	reference
Moderate	68 (22.7)	0.0377 (-0.0270, 0.1024)
High	86 (28.8)	0.0176 (-0.0440, 0.0792)
Very High	62 (20.7)	0.0436 (-0.0262, 0.1134)
Social and Economic Opportunity		
Continuous	27 (34)	-0.0001 (-0.0011, 0.0009)
Categories, n(%)		
Very Low	107 (35.8)	reference
Low	96 (32.1)	0.0051 (-0.0507, 0.0609)
Moderate	42 (14.0)	-0.0070 (-0.0800, 0.0659)
High/ Very High	54 (18.1)	-0.0053 (-0.0772, 0.0666)
Average annual ambient residential $PM_{2.5}$ ($\mu g/m^3$)	11.8 (2.5)	-0.02 (-0.04, -0.01)*

Abbreviations: PM2.5, Particulate Matter 2.5 μm; IQR, interquartile range; CI, Confidence Interval; COI, Child Opportunity Index.

All models adjusted for child age, gender, caregiver education, and child race.

* denotes statistically significant at $p<0.05$.

The association between average annual residential $PM_{2.5}$ exposure and TL did not differ significantly by COI or COI domains (p-interaction>0.10). Interaction plots revealed that the regression line slopes for associations between average annual $PM_{2.5}$ and TL increased as census tract Educational opportunity domain scores decreased (see figure 3).

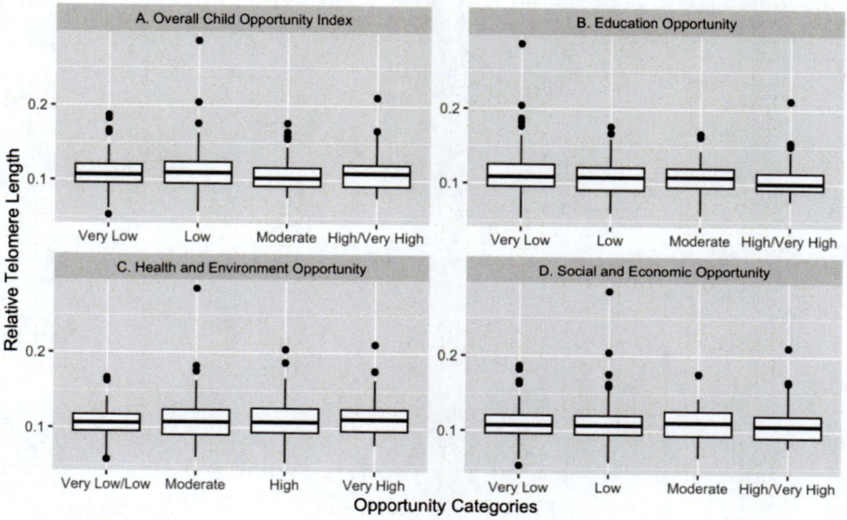

Figure 2. Distribution of telomere length by child opportunity index. Telomere length did not differ by A. overall Child Opportunity Index ($p = 0.68$), B. Education opportunity ($p = 0.22$), C. Health and Environment opportunity ($p = 0.74$), or D. Social and Economic opportunity ($p = 0.93$).

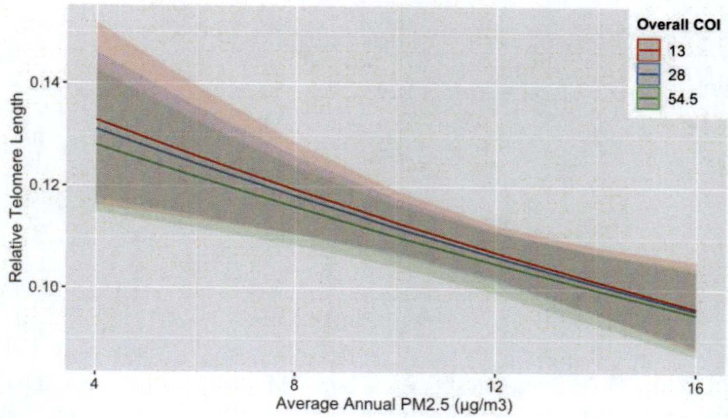

a.

Figure 3. (Continued).

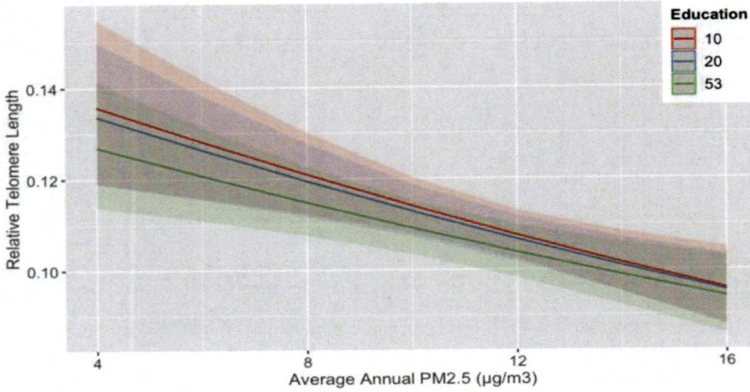

b.

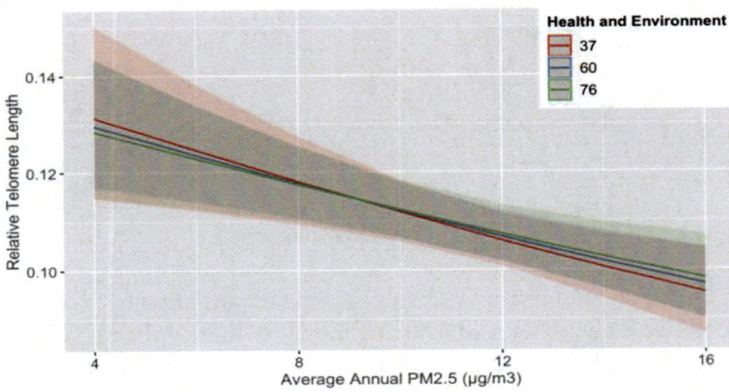

c.

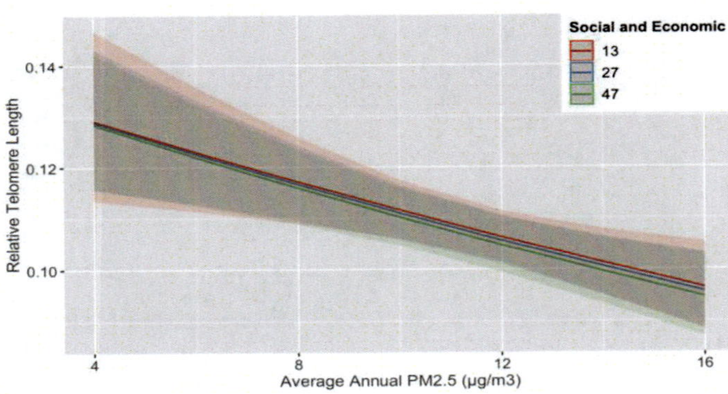

d.

Figure 3. Associations between average annual $PM_{2.5}$ and telomere length by child opportunity index. Multivariable linear regression results adjusted for age, gender, race and ethnicity, and caregiver education. Lines represent regression results stratified by 25th, 50th, and 75th percentile cutoffs of continuous neighborhood opportunity index. Associations did not differ by a. overall Child Opportunity Index (COI) ($p = 0.82$), b. Education opportunity ($p = 0.65$), c. Health and Environment opportunity ($p = 0.63$), or d. Social and Economic opportunity ($p = 0.91$).

In sensitivity analyses, our multivariable regression between COI and TL results remained null after controlling for early-life adversities. Correlation tests revealed that neither continuous COI and early-life adversities (r = -0.02, 95% CI: -0.16, 0.12) nor continuous COI domain scores (Education: r= -0.02, 95% CI: -0.16, 0.12 ; Health and Environment: r = 0.07, 95% CI: -0.08, 0.20; Social and Economic: r = -0.05, 95% CI: -0.19, 0.09) and early-life adversities were significantly correlated. Early-life adversities were also not significantly correlated with TL (r = -0.08, 95% CI: -0.22, 0.06).

Discussion

Based on prior literature that air pollution is associated with shorter TL and favorable neighborhood environments is associated with TL, we sought to examine associations between neighborhood child opportunity and air pollution exposure with TL among children to identify specific neighborhood assets that could buffer the adverse association between air pollution and TL. As expected, chronic residential $PM_{2.5}$ exposure was associated with shorter TL among children in our study. Our study did not find significant associations between the COI, an objective measure of neighborhood assets and opportunities relevant to children's health, and telomere length, a biomarker of physiological aging, among children. We also did not find differences in the adverse association between $PM_{2.5}$ and telomere length by COI domains. While the findings in this study were null, this is the first study to examine the impact of a comprehensive index of neighborhood assets on TL among children.

One potential explanation may be that the children studied (ages 1-11 years) were too young for neighborhood effects on TL to manifest, given the cumulative nature of telomere attrition across the lifecourse (40). While we did not observe associations at baseline, the relationships should be examined longitudinally to capture change in telomere attrition over time and to also identify critical windows of susceptibility to the neighborhood environment.

Our study results align with a systematic review that found limited evidence for an association between objective neighborhood socioeconomic characteristics and TL among adults (9). However, the COI assessed in our study captured objective measures of neighborhood characteristics, such as number of early childhood development centers, percentage of green space, and percentage of employed adults (1), whereas the majority of prior associations in other studies were between subjective, perceived neighborhood characteristics and TL among adults (9).

Theall et al. (21) did however find an effect of adverse environmental factors on TL among children between the ages of 5-16 years. They found that the density of liquor and convenience stores and rates of violent crime and domestic violence within 500 meters of children's residences were inversely associated with TL (21). This finding suggests that proximity to neighborhood exposures may mediate relationships with TL. We were not able to assess the role of proximity to neighborhood exposures given that the COI child opportunity measures were assigned to participant residential census tracts at baseline. This finding may also suggest the types of severe neighborhood stressors (e.g., violence and substance use) that are most impactful on TL in children. Our group's prior work supports this by finding an interaction of Social Context early-life adversities, which includes perceived neighborhood violence, on the inverse association between chronic PM2.5 exposure and TL in this study population (29). Additionally, our sensitivity analyses revealed that early-life adversities, such as abuse, neglect, household challenges, and social determinants of health, were not correlated with COI or TL. These findings suggest that early-life adversities are not mediating or confounding relationships between neighborhood opportunities and TL, again, because it is still too soon to observe effects of cumulative stress on TL.

Although the COI assessed in our study spanned multiple domains of neighborhood resources, there are likely additional community resources and assets pertinent to health that are not measured, such as participation in religious gatherings (41). Future qualitative assessments of neighborhoods are warranted to explore the perception of and access to neighborhood opportunities as a mediator between census-tract neighborhood opportunity and TL. We did find some trends towards neighborhood opportunities buffering the relationship between $PM_{2.5}$ and shorter TL, where the adverse association between $PM_{2.5}$ and TL seemed to be of lower magnitude for children living in neighborhoods with greater opportunity (see figure 2). However, none of these interactions were statistically significant.

Given the homogeneity of the study population in terms of socioeconomic status and that participants were mostly from historically marginalized racial and ethnic groups, there is a possibility that the study was underrepresented at levels of higher neighborhood opportunity thus not allowing for comparison across a broad range of neighborhood opportunity levels. Lack of neighborhood opportunity was prevalent in the study population, as 33.4% and 28.8% of the children in this study lived in census tracts that were categorized as "Very Low" and "Low" in opportunity, respectively. Given that the COI categories were constructed such that all census tracts in California were categorized into quintiles ("Very low" census tracts in the lowest quintile of COI, and "very high" census tracts in the highest quintile of COI), participants in our study were overrepresented in census tracts with lower COI scores.

Breaking the cycle of children's environmental health disparities by identifying potential resources to mitigate the harmful effects of $PM_{2.5}$ among children living in under-resourced neighborhoods calls for additional longitudinal research assessing the impact on older children and adolescents across levels of COI (ranging from "Very Low" to "Very High"), their neighborhood perceptions, proximity to neighborhood exposures, and community-partnered interventions.

Strengths

A major strength of this study was that the study population consisted of predominantly non-Hispanic Black and Latinx children, a population with disproportionate exposure to air pollution and neighborhood disadvantage. Targeted recruitment of this study population was intentional to inform interventions among a highly stressed population.

Limitations

This current study design was cross-sectional, thus we are unable to establish causality or temporality between neighborhood environment and TL. Additionally, the children in our study were young, thus it may be too soon to detect long-term relationships with TL. Longitudinal studies that measure TL across childhood are needed to more precisely characterize the effects of neighborhood exposures. The study was also likely underpowered to detect associations between COI and TL and multiplicative interaction between COI and $PM_{2.5}$. Utilizing minimum detectable effect levels derived from prior studies on objective neighborhood characteristics and TL among children and adults (12, 21), this study has a 5% power to detect an estimate of $\beta = .006$ and a 10% power to detect an estimate of $\beta = .04$. To detect an interaction effect estimate of 0.001, this study has 10% power (42). Additional power calculations showed that having an 80% powered study would require at least 4,902 participants. However, we were still able to detect the inverse association between $PM_{2.5}$ and TL; future studies should continue these analyses with larger sample sizes, especially with greater representation in census tracts with greater opportunity levels. We also acknowledge that the presence of opportunities in each census tract does not necessarily equate to access or usage by the study participants. Average annual $PM_{2.5}$ estimates were assigned to residential addresses provided at study baseline, thus it is possible that the participants moved during this time, resulting in exposure misclassification and a bias towards the null.

Conclusion

Neighborhood opportunity measured using the COI was not found to be associated with modification of TL among children ages 1-11 in this study. Future research that is longitudinal, among older children and adolescents, across a wider range of neighborhood opportunity and that assesses children's neighborhood perception and proximity to exposures is warranted to further identify resilience factors that may buffer the adverse association between air pollution and telomere length. Future directions include measuring TL in this cohort at a later time.

Acknowledgments

The preparation for this project and manuscript review was supported by the Break the Cycle of Health Disparities Program of the Southeast PEHSU at Emory University and Break the Cycle of Health Disparities, Inc. Austin Le was supported by the Kirk R. Smith Memorial Fellowship.

References

[1] Noelke C, McArdle N, Baek M, Huntington N, Huber R, Hardy E, et al. Child Opportunity Index 2.0 Technical Documentation [Internet]. 2020. URL: diversitydatakids.org/researchlibrary/research-brief/how-we-built-it.

[2] Beck AF, Huang B, Wheeler K, Lawson NR, Kahn RS, Riley CL. The Child Opportunity Index and disparities in pediatric asthma hospitalizations across one Ohio Metropolitan Area, 2011-2013. J Pediatrics 2017;190:200-6.

[3] Aris IM, Rifas-Shiman SL, Jimenez MP, Li LJ, Hivert MF, Oken E, et al. Neighborhood Child Opportunity Index and adolescent cardiometabolic risk. Pediatrics 2021;147(2):e2020018903.

[4] Vaiserman A, Krasnienkov D. Telomere length as a marker of biological age: State-of-the-Art, open issues, and future perspectives. Front Genetics 2021;11:630186.

[5] Herrmann M, Pusceddu I, März W, Herrmann W. Telomere biology and age-related diseases. Clin Chem Lab Med 2018;56(8):1210–22.

[6] Aviv A, Anderson JJ, Shay JW. Mutations, cancer and the telomere length paradox. Trends Cancer 2017;3(4):253–8.

[7] Shay JW, Wright WE. Role of telomeres and telomerase in cancer. Semin Cancer Biol 2011;21(6):349–53.

[8] Turner KJ, Vasu V, Griffin DK. Telomere biology and human phenotype. Cells 2019;8(1):73.

[9] Coimbra BM, Carvalho CM, van Zuiden M, Williamson RE, Ota VK, Mello AF, et al. The impact of neighborhood context on telomere length: A systematic review. Health Place 2022;74:102746.

[10] Troxel WM, Madrigano J, Haas AC, Dubowitz T, Rosso AL, Prather AA, et al. Examining the cross-sectional association between neighborhood conditions, discrimination, and telomere Length in a predominantly African American sample. J Racial Ethnic Health Disparities 2023;10:3159-67.

[11] Massey DS, Wagner B, Donnelly L, McLanahan S, Brooks-Gunn J, Garfinkel I, et al. Neighborhood disadvantage and telomere length: Results from the Fragile Families Study. Russell Sage Foundation J Soc Sci 2018 Apr 1;4(4):28–42.

[12] Powell-Wiley TM, Gebreab SY, Claudel SE, Ayers C, Andrews MR, Adu-Brimpong J, et al. The relationship between neighborhood socioeconomic deprivation and telomere length: The 1999–2002 National Health and Nutrition Examination Survey. SSM Populat Health 2020;10:100517.

[13] Alexeeff SE, Schaefer CA, Kvale MN, Shan J, Blackburn EH, Risch N, et al. Telomere length and socioeconomic status at neighborhood and individual levels among 80,000 adults in the Genetic Epidemiology Research on Adult Health and Aging cohort. Environ Epidemiol 2019;3(3):e049.

[14] Lynch SM, Mitra N, Ravichandran K, Mitchell J, Spangler E, Zhou W, et al. Telomere length and neighborhood circumstances: Evaluating biological response to unfavorable exposures. Cancer Epidemiol Biomark Prev 2017;26(4):553–60.

[15] Gebreab SY, Riestra P, Gaye A, Khan RJ, Xu R, Davis AR, et al. Perceived neighborhood problems are associated with shorter telomere length in African American women. Psychoneuroendocrinol 2016;69:90–7.

[16] Thierry AD. Association between telomere length and neighborhood characteristics by race and region in US midlife and older adults. Health Place 2020;62:102272.

[17] Park M, Verhoeven JE, Cuijpers P, Reynolds III CF, Penninx BWJH. Where you live may make you old: The association between perceived poor neighborhood quality and leukocyte telomere length. PLoS One 2015;10(6):e0128460.

[18] Needham BL, Carroll JE, Diez Roux AV, Fitzpatrick AL, Moore K, Seeman TE. Neighborhood characteristics and leukocyte telomere length: The Multi-Ethnic Study of Atherosclerosis. Health Place 2014;28:167–72.

[19] Ellaway A, Dundas R, Robertson T, Shiels PG. More miles on the clock: Neighbourhood stressors are associated with telomere length in a longitudinal study. PLoS One 2019;14(3):e0214380.

[20] Theall KP, Brett ZH, Shirtcliff EA, Dunn EC, Drury SS. Neighborhood disorder and telomeres: Connecting children's exposure to community level stress and cellular response. Soc Sci Med 2013;85:50–8.

[21] Theall KP, Shirtcliff EA, Dismukes AR, Wallace M, Drury SS. Association between neighborhood violence and biological stress in children. JAMA Pediatrics 2017;171(1):53–60.

[22] Miri M, de Prado-Bert P, Alahabadi A, Najafi ML, Rad A, Moslem A, et al. Association of greenspace exposure with telomere length in preschool children. Environ Pollution 2020;266:115228.

[23] Brown R, Hailu EM, Needham BL, Roux AD, Seeman TE, Lin J, et al. Neighborhood social environment and changes in leukocyte telomere length: The Multi-Ethnic Study of Atherosclerosis (MESA). Health Place 2021;67:102488.

[24] Morello-Frosch R, Zuk M, Jerrett M, Shamasunder B, Kyle AD. Understanding the cumulative impacts of inequalities in environmental health: implications for policy. Health Aff (Millwood) 2011;30(5):879–87.

[25] Clark LP, Millet DB, Marshall JD. Changes in transportation-related air pollution exposures by race-ethnicity and socioeconomic status: Outdoor nitrogen dioxide in the United States in 2000 and 2010. Environ Health Perspect 2017;125(9):097012.

[26] Williams DR, Priest N, Anderson NB. Understanding associations among race, socioeconomic status, and health: Patterns and prospects. Health Psychol 2016;35(4):407–11.

[27] Misra S, Kwon SC, Abraído-Lanza AF, Chebli P, Trinh-Shevrin C, Yi SS. Structural racism and immigrant health in the United States. Health Educ Behav 2021;48(3):332–41.

[28] Rubin IL, Geller RJ, Martinuzzi K, Howett M, Gitterman BA, Wells L, et al. Break the cycle of environmental health disparities: An ecological framework. Int Public Health J 2017;9(2):115–27.

[29] de la Rosa R, Le A, Holm S, et al. Associations Between Early-Life Adversity, Ambient Air Pollution, and Telomere Length in Children. Psychosomatic Medicine. Published online February 12, 2024:10.1097/PSY.0000000000001276.

[30] Lee EY, Oh SS, White MJ, Eng CS, Elhawary JR, Borrell LN, et al. Ambient air pollution, asthma drug response, and telomere length in African American youth. J Allergy Clin Immunol 2019;144(3):839-845.e10.

[31] Hautekiet P, Nawrot TS, Janssen BG, Martens DS, De Clercq EM, Dadvand P, et al. Child buccal telomere length and mitochondrial DNA content as biomolecular markers of ageing in association with air pollution. Environ Int 2021;147:106332.

[32] Clemente DBP, Vrijheid M, Martens DS, Bustamante M, Chatzi L, Danileviciute A, et al. Prenatal and childhood traffic-related air pollution exposure and telomere length in European children: The HELIX Project. Environmental Health Perspect 2019;127(8):087001.

[33] Moslem A, Rad A, de Prado Bert P, Alahabadi A, Ebrahimi Aval H, Miri M, et al. Association of exposure to air pollution and telomere length in preschool children. Sci Total Environ 2020;722:137933.

[34] Thakur N, Hessler D, Koita K, Ye M, Benson M, Gilgoff R, et al. Pediatrics adverse childhood experiences and related life events screener (PEARLS) and health in a safety-net practice. Child Abuse Negl 2020;108:104685.

[35] van Donkelaar A, Martin RV, Li C, Burnett RT. Regional estimates of chemical composition of fine particulate matter using a combined geoscience-statistical method with information from satellites, models, and monitors. Environ Sci Technol 2019;53(5):2595–611.

[36] Cawthon RM. Telomere measurement by quantitative PCR. Nucleic Acids Res 2002;30(10):e47.

[37] O'Callaghan NJ, Fenech M. A quantitative PCR method for measuring absolute telomere length. Biol Proced Online 2011;13:3.

[38] Thiese MS, Ronna B, Ott U. P value interpretations and considerations. J Thorac Dis 2016;8(9):E928–31.

[39] RStudio Team. RStudio: Integrated development for R [Internet]. Boston, MA: RStudio, PBC, 2020. URL: http://www.rstudio.com/.

[40] Collins K. The biogenesis and regulation of telomerase holoenzymes. Nat Rev Mol Cell Biol 2006;7(7):484–94.

[41] Anyfantakis D, Symvoulakis EK, Lionis CD. Religiosity, well-being and 'slowing down' Ageing damage: A literature review. Cureus 2020;12(8):e9910.

[42] Baranger DAA, Finsaas MC, Goldstein BL, Vize CE, Lynam DR, Olino TM. Tutorial: Power analyses for interaction effects in cross-sectional regressions. Adv Methods Pract Psychol Sci 2023;6(3):25152459231187531.

Chapter 5

The relationship between race and access to public water and sewer service in Halifax County, North Carolina

Banks Grubbs, BSPH*
and Jacqueline MacDonald Gibson, PhD
Department of Civil, Construction, and Environmental Engineering, North Carolina State University, Raleigh, North Carolina, United States of America

Numerous studies have shown that Black communities on the fringes of Southern towns and cities in the United States have been systematically denied access to critical infrastructure such as public water and sewer services. This research investigates the relationship between race and access to these services within the six extraterritorial jurisdictions (ETJs) of Halifax County, North Carolina. Utilizing multivariate logistic regressions, the relationship between the proportion of Black people living in a census block and the odds of a residence in that block having public water or sewer access was estimated. Significant negative relationships were identified between the proportion of Black people per census block and odds of access to public water in the ETJs of Roanoke Rapids (OR = 0.24, $p = 0.0237$) and Littleton (OR = 0.025, $p = 0.0162$), and the odds of access to sewer service in the ETJs of Roanoke Rapids (OR = 0.04, $p<0.001$), Littleton (OR = 0.027, $p = 0.0162$), and Scotland Neck (OR = 0.259, $p = 0.032$). These results suggest that predominantly Black communities in these ETJs are less likely to have access to public water and sewer services. People who do not have access to these services are more likely to rely on private wells and septic systems, which are associated with increased exposure to contaminants like lead and disease-causing microorganisms. Therefore, these excluded communities are potentially more likely to be exposed to harmful environmental

* Corresponding Author's E-mail: bagrubbs@ncsu.edu

In: Neighborhoods: Impact on Child Health and Development
Editors: I Leslie Rubin and Joav Merrick
ISBN: 979-8-89530-834-9

contaminants and to experience related negative health outcomes, contributing to a cycle of environmental health disparities.

Introduction

Access to public water and sewer service has been shown to reduce exposure to a variety of harmful environmental contaminants and reduce the incidence of related diseases (1). However, numerous studies have shown that Black communities on the fringes of rural southern towns have been historically denied access to these utilities, a pattern sometimes referred to as municipal underbounding (2–9). Municipal underbounding is often achieved through the use of discriminatory zoning and annexation practices, such as selectively expanding corporate boundaries to exclude communities of color, or through the use of extraterritorial jurisdictions (ETJs), which are common in North Carolina.

ETJs are powerful tools that allow municipalities to designate areas up to three miles outside of their borders for future annexation (10). Within ETJs, municipal governments are granted power over zoning and subdivision ordinances, housing and building codes, and community development regulations. However, there is no obligation for municipalities to extend public services into ETJs, and residents are not guaranteed the right to vote in municipal elections (11). Historically, many municipalities have drawn ETJs around Black communities located just outside of their borders. However, instead of making improvements to these areas and eventually annexing them, the municipalities use their newfound regulatory power to maintain control over these communities without needing to fund expensive utility expansion projects and other basic amenities.

This has been documented in many North Carolina towns, such as Mebane (2, 3), Pinehurst (9), and the eight towns studied in Parnell et al. (4). Mebane is a rural majority-white town that has strategically drawn its borders to exclude the four nearby Black communities. These communities appear to have been intentionally excluded from the town and systematically denied access to public water and sewer services. Despite their proximity to the town, their long-term residence in the ETJ, and their many petitions, these communities have yet to be annexed, though many of the predominantly white neighborhoods nearby have been (2, 3). Similarly, several Black communities lie within the ETJ of Pinehurst, a wealthy town known for its large golf resort. Just as in Mebane, Pinehurst seems to have systematically excluded communities of color from the town boundaries and intentionally denied them access to basic amenities (9). Patterns such as these are commonplace in the South. This research seeks to determine if these patterns are also present in the ETJs of Halifax County, North Carolina.

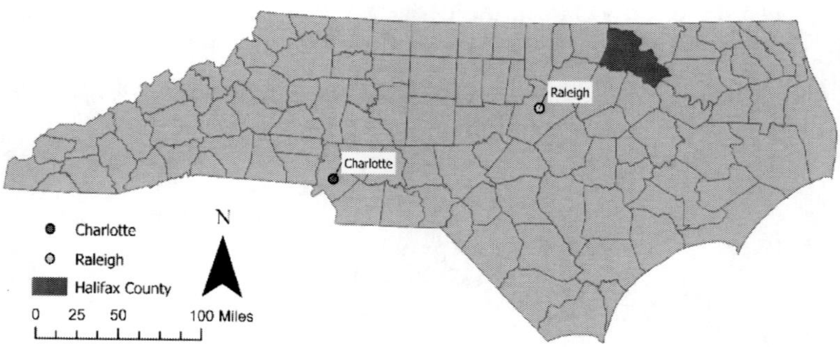

Figure 1. Map of North Carolina highlighting Halifax County.

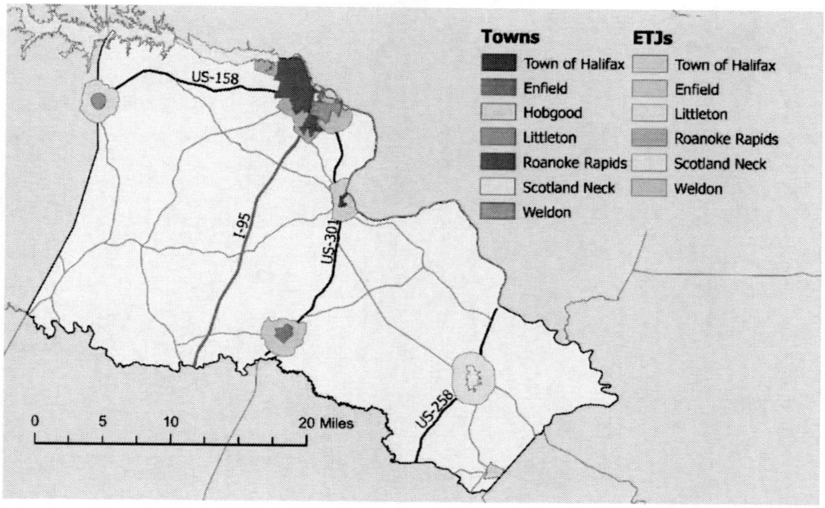

Figure 2. Halifax County, North Carolina, its towns, ETJs, and major roadways.

Halifax County background and history

Halifax County (see figure 1) is a rural county in North Carolina with an estimated population of 47,848 people (12). Of the seven municipalities in Halifax County, six have extraterritorial jurisdictions (see figure 2).

Halifax County, and much of the surrounding land, was originally the territory of the Tuscarora people (13). This indigenous community was driven out of the area in the early 18th century by English colonizers. These colonizers quickly established plantations where they forced enslaved people to produce a variety of crops in the fertile soil along the Roanoke River (14). The county quickly became an important trade center, with an economy relying heavily on this agricultural enslavement; in the 1860 census a total of 10,349 enslaved people and 2,452 "free colored" people were recorded living in the county, almost double the white population of 6,641 (15).

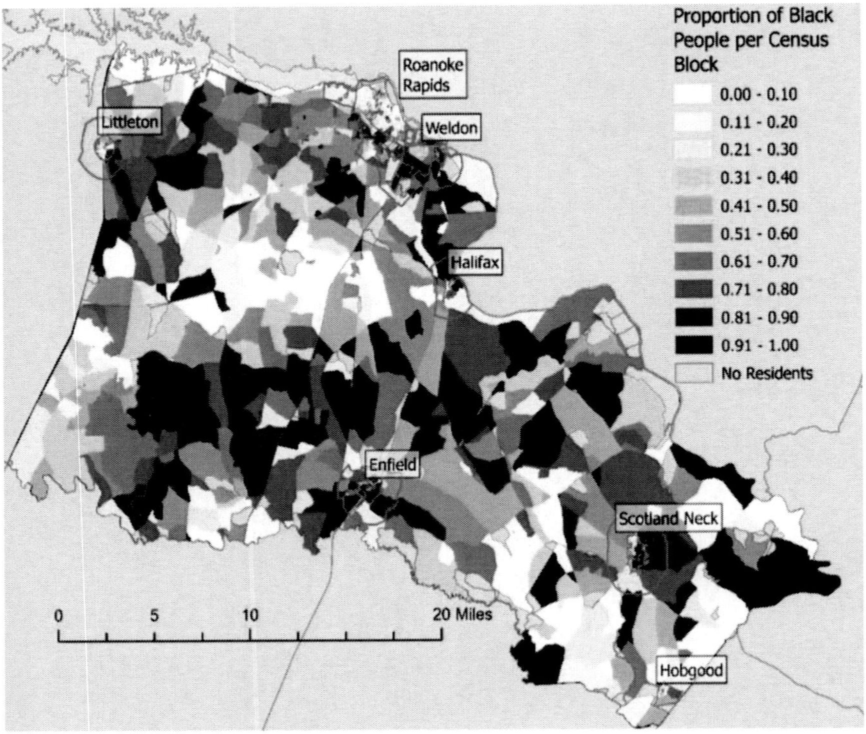

Figure 3. Proportion of Black people per census block in Halifax County.

According to the 2020 census, a majority of Halifax County's residents still identify as Black or African American (53.3%) (12). However, many of the towns are predominantly white, with Black communities seemingly relegated to the fringes or just outside of the town border (see figure 3). This trend is well documented in other small southern towns, and is a product of both historic land ownership patterns and the settlement patterns of Black migrants in the late 1960s and 70s (16). The exclusion of these communities from modern-day borders echoes the exclusion seen in other towns, such as Mebane and Pinehurst. Excluded communities are deprived of political and social power and are often denied access to important public health services like public water and sewer systems.

Importance of public water and sewer service

Access to public water and sewer service is important for public health, as these services have been shown to reduce exposure to a variety of harmful environmental contaminants (1). People who do not have access to these services usually rely on private wells and septic systems as an alternative. However, private wells and septic systems are associated with an increased risk of exposure to harmful environmental contaminants that can cause a variety of negative health outcomes (1, 17, 18), especially in populated areas such as residential neighborhoods within ETJs.

Drinking water provided by public water systems is treated to meet a variety of regulatory safety standards set by the United States Environmental Protection Agency (EPA), as mandated by the Safe Drinking Water Act. Those without access to public water often rely on private wells for their drinking water, which are not regulated by the Safe Drinking Water Act. Newly constructed wells in North Carolina must be tested once before use, but older wells do not have this requirement (19). Therefore, the well owners are solely responsible for the maintenance, testing, and treatment of their water. Unfortunately, the costs of these services can be prohibitively high, and research has shown that many well users do not know the potential risks of untreated water and do not know how to test or treat their water (20). Due in part to these barriers, private wells are recognized as a potential source of exposure to a variety of chemical and biological contaminants that can lead to adverse health effects like acute gastrointestinal illness and developmental impairment (18, 21).

Access to sewer services is also important for public health. In North Carolina, the main alternative to sewer service is a septic system. When properly installed and maintained these systems adequately treat human fecal waste and pose little health risk. However, they are not always installed properly, and maintenance can be complicated and expensive. This can lead to users poorly maintaining their systems, resulting in failure (22). Failing septic systems can be a major source of fecal exposure (23, 24), and proximity to a high concentration of septic systems is associated with increased gastrointestinal illnesses like viral and bacterial diarrhea (17).

In this study, we seek to understand the relationship between race and the odds of access to public water and sewer service within the six ETJs in Halifax County. By identifying and quantifying utility access disparities, we can better understand the impact of historical racial discrimination on modern-day health inequities and identify opportunities to extend utilities to these marginalized communities.

Our study

Population data from the 2020 decennial census at the census block level and a shapefile representing each census block was obtained from the US Census Bureau. These records were then joined based on their block numbers, and the population density and proportion of Black people living in each block was calculated. A person was considered Black if they described themselves as either "Black or African American" in any capacity (i.e., if an individual identified as multiple races, including "Black or African American," they were considered to be Black for this analysis).

Extraterritorial jurisdictions and geographical data

The Halifax County Tax Administration office provided shapefiles denoting town/municipal borders, the county border, and county-maintained roads. Notably, neither the Halifax County government nor most towns within the county maintain a shapefile for extraterritorial jurisdictions. Therefore, these shapefiles were created manually based on zoning maps obtained from each town.

ETJs were selected as the extent of the analysis for two main reasons. First, in NC, the limits of an ETJ generally cannot extend beyond three miles from the town borders, and can only extend one mile beyond the border if the population of the municipality is less than 10,000 people (10). Therefore, all parcels within ETJs are inherently close to the nearby town (where a vast majority of parcels are expected to have public water and sewer service). Second, ETJs are meant to identify areas for future annexation by the parent municipality. Assuming residents of the municipality have access to public water and sewer services, it is expected that municipalities will eventually extend these utilities to ETJ residents. This expectation is not held for people who simply live near a town but not with an ETJ, as there is no expectation of potential future annexation.

Tax data

Tax records for 2020 and a shapefile denoting every tax parcel in the county were provided by the Halifax County Tax Administration office. The shapefile and tax records were then joined based on their parcel ID number, producing a spatial dataset of every tax parcel and its taxable value, livable area, municipal zoning, address, owner address, and utility connections.

After processing the census and tax records, every tax parcel was joined with its census block based on the location of its centroid. This added two data points to each tax parcel: the population density and the proportion of Black people in the census block.

Estimating ownership status

Homeownership is a potentially important marker of generational wealth. Therefore, we estimated the owner/tenant status of each residential parcel within the ETJs. This was done by comparing the owner's address, as listed in the tax records, with the address of the tax parcel. If the addresses matched, the parcel was considered to be occupied by the owner. Otherwise, the parcel was considered to be occupied by a tenant.

Distance from the Roanoke Rapids Wastewater Treatment Plant

To estimate the relative cost of extending sewer lines to the parcels in the Roanoke Rapids ETJ, the most efficient (least-cost) path between each parcel and the Roanoke Rapids Sanitary District Wastewater Treatment Plant (WWTP) was estimated utilizing ArcGIS Pro (Version: 3.1.2). To generate the least-cost path, we converted a shapefile of state-maintained roads into a cost surface raster with a 30m resolution. Each pixel was then assigned a cost, meant to represent the likelihood of a sewer line being routed through said area. Pixels that represent roads were given a cost of 1 and all other pixels were given a cost of 5, to represent a significant increase in development cost. These values represent that sewer lines are often built along roads, rather than through private or developed land, but that it is still possible to route lines through non-road surfaces. Then, for each parcel, the path with the lowest accumulated cost was calculated. This cost was then appended to each parcel as a new variable representing the relative cost to establish a connection from the parcel to the WWTP.

The effect of including this variable in the regression was then investigated and the correlation between the proportion of Black people per census block and the relative distance between parcels and the WWTP was calculated.

Statistical methods

Statistical analysis was conducted with R (25), RStudio (26), and the tidyverse package (27). Of the initial 39,305 parcels imported, only 1,752 remained after evaluating for exclusion criteria. Parcels were excluded if they were not in an ETJ, were not an apartment complex or residentially zoned, were listed as having no livable area, or were in an unpopulated census block.

Logistic regressions

Logistic regressions for public water and sewer access were conducted independently on each of the six ETJs. It should be noted that each ETJ was treated as an independent population, as the social and historical context of each ETJ's municipality is different. This important context would be masked if all ETJs were treated as a single group. For each ETJ, two regressions were conducted – one where the outcome variable was access to public water and the other where the outcome variable was access to public sewer. Both regressions had the same independent predictor variables: the proportion of Black people in the census block, the taxable value of the parcel (USD), the population density of the census block (people per sq. km.), and the estimated ownership status (owner or tenant). These variables are summarized and compared in table 1.

Table 1. Summary information for each town and ETJ

Characteristic	Enfield		Hobgood		Littleton		Roanoke Rapids	
	Municipality	ETJ	Municipality	ETJ	Municipality	ETJ	Municipality	ETJ
Number of Residential Parcels*	769	217	157	—	274	143	5260	772
Median Taxable Value of Parcel (USD)*	$45,100	$61,100	$33,300	—	$60,050	$40,000	$76,150	$105,750
Average Population Density (per sq. km.)+	797	486	467	—	314	250	1235	627
Average Proportion of Black People per Census Block+	0.805	0.759	0.19	—	0.37	0.71	0.29	0.35

Characteristic	Scotland Neck		Town of Halifax		Weldon	
	Municipality	ETJ	Municipality	ETJ	Municipality	ETJ
Number of Residential Parcels*	848	214	111	130	657	276
Median Taxable Value of Parcel (USD)*	$40,000	$53,250	$63,600	$44,550	$49,100	$31,750
Average Population Density (per sq. km.)+	591	69	364	228	252	516
Average Proportion of Black People per Census Block+	0.81	0.41	0.20	0.62	0.83	0.74

* Tax parcel resolution

\+ Census block resolution

Table 2. Regression results for sewer service access

Regression Results: Public Sewer Access by Town

	Roanoke Rapids (n = 772)		Enfield (n = 217)		Town of Halifax (n = 130)	
Characteristic	**Estimate**	**p-value**	**Estimate**	**p-value**	**Estimate**	**p-value**
Proportion Black	-3.216	**<0.001**	1.156	0.152	2.294	0.060
Tax Value	-2.98e-06	**0.006**	-4.85e-06	0.196	3.21e-07	0.947
Population Density	0.002	**<0.001**	-9.68e-04	0.167	0.003	**<0.001**
Ownership Status						
Owner	—		—		—	
Tenant	0.386	**0.024**	0.512	0.132	1.639	0.139

	Weldon (n = 276)		Scotland Neck (n = 214)		Littleton (n = 144)	
Characteristic	**Estimate**	**p-value**	**Estimate**	**p-value**	**Estimate**	**p-value**
Proportion Black	-0.485	0.627	-1.352	**0.032**	-3.606	**0.016**
Tax Value	-8.37e-06	0.159	2.38e-06	0.343	-1.38e-05	**0.025**
Population Density	0.009	**<0.001**	0.004	0.104	0.006	**0.002**
Ownership Status						
Owner	—		—		—	
Tenant	-0.543	0.268	0.396	0.246	1.313	**0.018**

Table 3. Regression results for sewer service access

Regression Results: Public Water Access by Town

	Roanoke Rapids (n = 772)		Enfield (n = 217)		Town of Halifax (n = 130)	
Characteristic	**Estimate**	**p-value**	**Estimate**	**p-value**	**Estimate**	**p-value**
Proportion Black	-1.426	**0.024**	-2.417	0.069	0.464	0.541
Tax Value	-5.06e-06	**<0.001**	-6.01e-06	0.253	-4.94e-06	0.178
Population Density	0.002	**<0.001**	0.002	0.248	2.28e-04	0.682
Ownership Status						
Owner	—		—		—	
Tenant	-0.481	0.087	0.259	0.557	1.238	**0.015**

	Weldon (n = 276)		Scotland Neck (n = 214)		Littleton (n = 144)	
Characteristic	**Estimate**	**p-value**	**Estimate**	**p-value**	**Estimate**	**p-value**
Proportion Black	1.736	0.112	-1.183	0.104	-3.705	**0.016**
Tax Value	-1.66e-05	**0.010**	-1.68e-06	0.524	-1.40e-05	**0.025**
Population Density	0.007	**0.002**	-0.001	0.579	0.009	**0.004**
Ownership Status						
Owner	—		—		—	
Tenant	-0.488	0.412	0.508	0.119	1.407	**0.014**

Taxable value includes the value of the land, built structures, and other miscellaneous improvements made to the parcel. This factor is a representation of the overall wealth of residents as well as the value of nearby properties and accounts for the suggestion that utilities could be preferentially expanded toward wealthier areas. If the proportion of Black people in the census block is found to have a significant effect when accounting for tax value, it suggests that race is a factor in access despite the effect of the wealth of the resident and the value of the property.

Population density represents the number of people per square kilometer of the census block. Including this factor accounts for the reasonable suggestion that municipalities will expand utilities to more densely populated areas before less densely populated ones in an effort to achieve the best cost-to-benefit ratio. By including this factor, we account for this – if the effect of the proportion of Black people per block is significant when considering the effect of population density, it suggests that there is an effect of race on access despite the effect of population density.

The estimated ownership status is intended to account for personal wealth, generational wealth, and the difference in political power between homeowners and tenants. Homeowners are more likely to hold some amount of generational wealth. This is especially important considering the history of Black Southerners, who have had significantly less time to accumulate this wealth and are less likely to have inherited a residence from their family.

Regression visualization

To visualize regression results, the odds of access to public water and sewer were estimated based on the regression equations. For each ETJ, the odds of access were predicted by holding the parcel tax value and population density at the median of the ETJ and by setting the ownership status, the reference value, then incrementally increasing the proportion of Black people per block by 0.05 from 0.00 to 1.00. This provided a visualization of how utility access is expected to change as the proportion of Black people per block increases in each ETJ.

Our findings

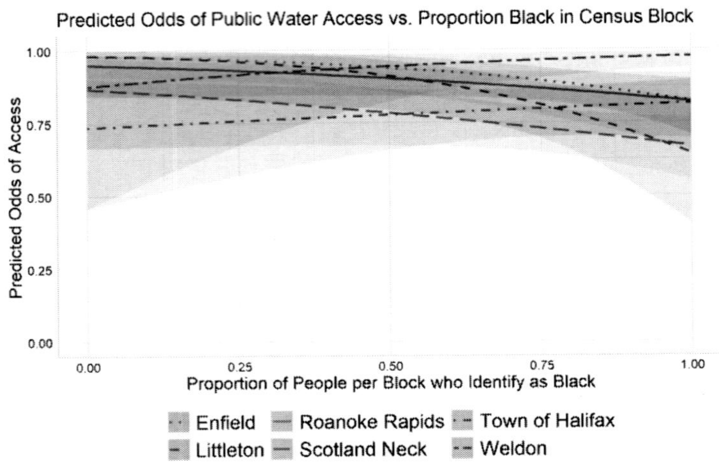

a.

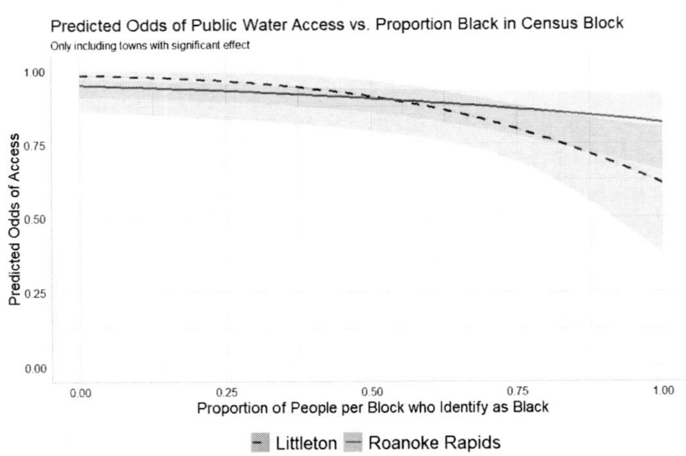

b.

Figure 4. Predicted odds of access to community water service as a function of the proportion of Black people per census block in each ETJ in Halifax County (a) and in the ETJs where a significant relationship was identified (b).

In the ETJs of Roanoke Rapids, Littleton, and Scotland Neck, significant negative associations were found between the proportion of Black people per census block and odds of a parcel in that block having utilities. The remaining ETJs (Enfield, Weldon, and the town of Halifax) did not appear to have a significant relationship. Regression results for sewer and public water access are given in table 2 and table 3, respectively. Additionally, to demonstrate the relative strengths of the association between race and utility access, the predicted odds of access to public water and sewer are shown in figure 4 and figure 5, respectively.

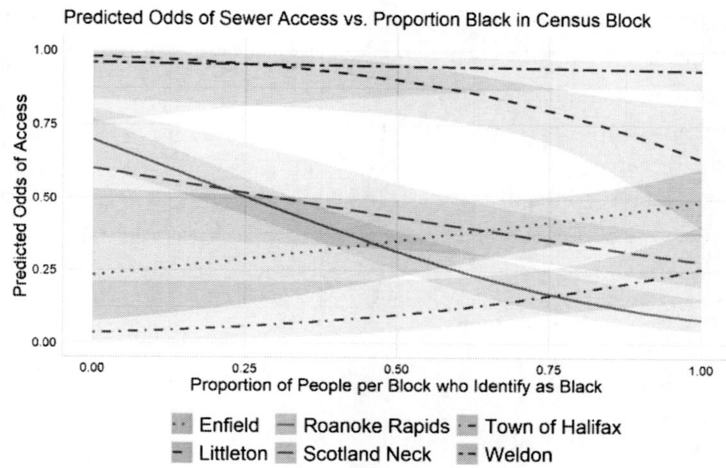

a.

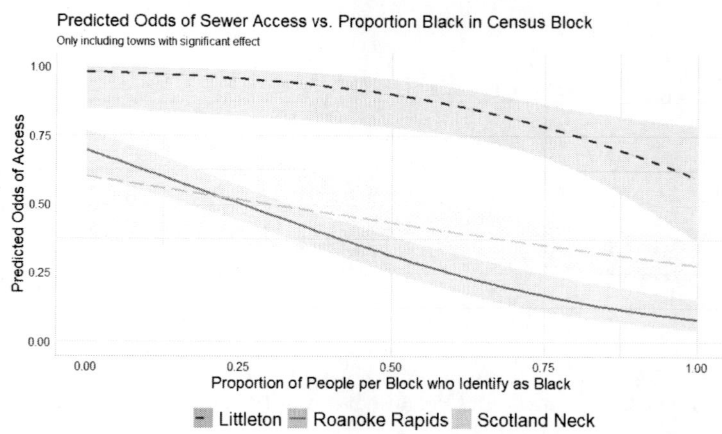

b.

Figure 5. Predicted odds of access to sewer service as a function of the proportion of Black people per census block in each ETJ in Halifax County 5a) and in the E TJs where a significant relationship was identified (b).

Roanoke Rapids

n Roanoke Rapids ETJ, as the proportion of Black people in a census block increases, the odds of access to public sewer and to public water service decreases significantly (sewer OR: 0.040, $p < 0.001$; public water OR: 0.24, $p = 0.024$). To demonstrate the strength of the effect, predicted odds of access to both public water and sewer were generated and plotted, as shown in figure 6. The relationship is strongest for sewer access – as demonstrated in the figure, as the proportion of Black people per census block increases from 0.0 to 1.0, the predicted odds of access to sewer (holding population density and tax value at their median, and ownership

Astatus as tenant) decreases from 0.69 (95CI: 0.61, 0.77) to 0.08 (95CI: 0.04, 0.16). Regarding water access, as the proportion of Black people per census block increases from 0.0 to 1.0 the predicted odds of access decreases from 0.95 (0.91, 0.97) to 0.82 (0.65, 0.92).

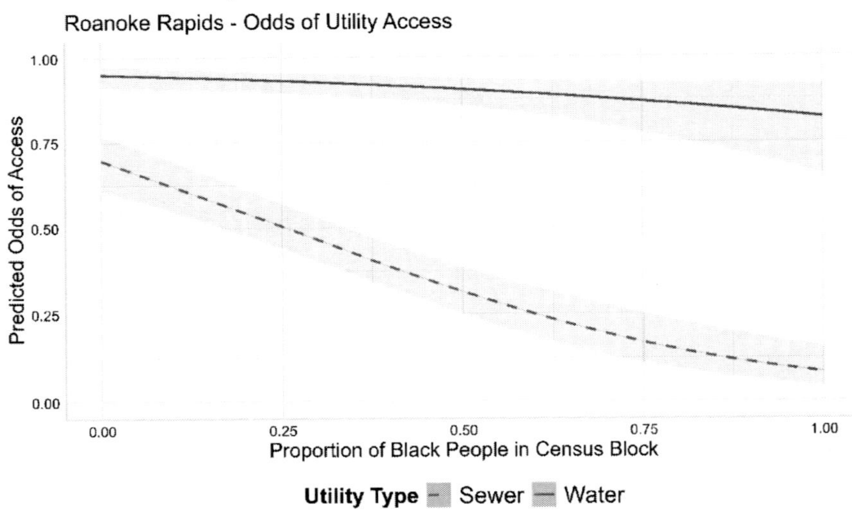

Figure 6. Predicted odds of access to sewer and community water service in the ETJ of Roanoke Rapids, as a function of the proportion of Black people in the census block.

We also considered how the effect of distance from the WWTP could affect these results, as it is expensive and time-consuming for municipalities to extend sewer lines. The correlation between the distance of a parcel from the WWTP and the proportion of Black people in the parcel's census block is strongly negatively correlated (-0.65). Additionally, when the distance variable is added to the regression, a strong positive correlation between distance and odds of sewer access was identified (OR: 1.81, $p<0.001$). Notably, when this variable is added, the effect of the proportion of Black people per block loses significance (p = 0.33). However, due to the strong correlation between these two variables, we suspect that the effect of the distance to the WWTP is masking the effect of the proportion of Black people per block.

Littleton

In the Littleton ETJ, as the proportion of Black people in a census block increases, the odds of access to sewer and to public water service decreases significantly (sewer OR: 0.035, p = 0.016; public water OR: 0.031, p = 0.016). To demonstrate the strength of the effect, predicted odds of access to both public water and sewer were generated and plotted, as shown in figure 7. As demonstrated in the figure, as the proportion of Black people per census block increases from 0.0 to 1.0, the predicted odds of access to public sewer decreases from 0.98 (0.83, 1.00) to 0.64 (0.40, 0.82), and the predicted odds of access to public water decreases from 0.98 (0.85, 1.00) to 0.64 (0.40, 0.83).

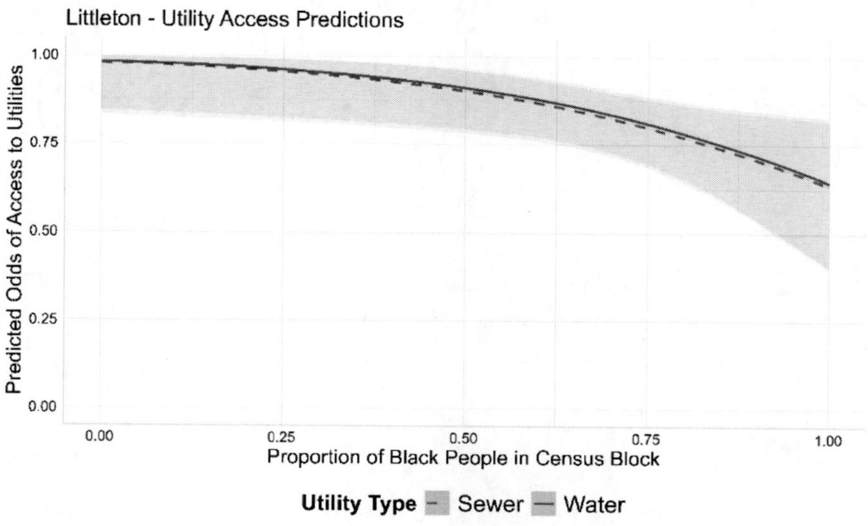

Figure 7. Predicted odds of access to sewer and community water service in the ETJ of Littleton, as a function of the proportion of Black people in the census block.

Scotland Neck

In the Scotland Neck ETJ, a significant relationship was identified between the proportion of Black people per block and odds of access to sewer (OR: 0.259, $p = 0.032$), but not public water (OR: 0.307, $p = 0.10$). As with the Roanoke Rapids and Littleton results, to demonstrate the strength of the effect, predicted odds of access to both public water and sewer were plotted, as shown in figure 8. This demonstrates that as the proportion of Black people in a census block increases from 0% to 100%, the predicted odds of access to sewer decreases from 0.60 (0.36, 0.80) to 0.28 (0.19, 0.39).

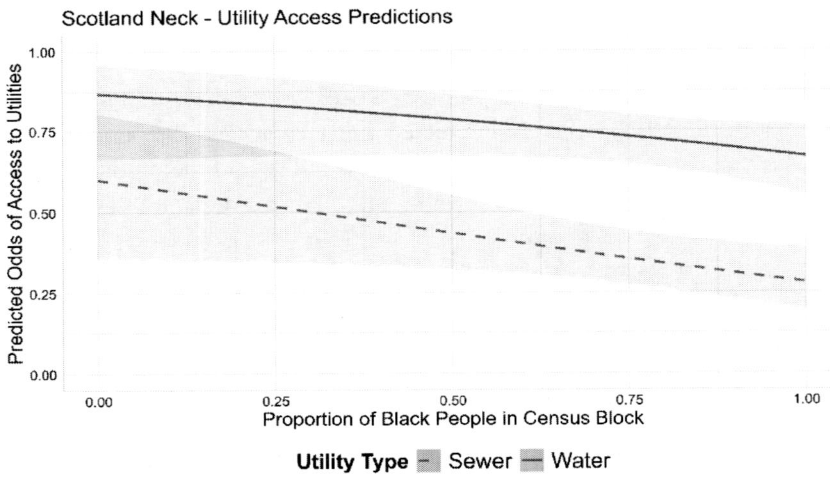

Figure 8. Predicted odds of access to sewer and community water service in the ETJ of Scotland Neck, as a function of the proportion of Black people in the census block.

Discussion

There appears to be a significant negative relationship between the proportion of Black people per census block in the ETJs of Roanoke Rapids, Littleton, and Scotland Neck and the odds of access to public water and sewer. This relationship remains significant when considering the effect of population density, the taxable value of the property, and the estimated ownership status of the residence. As reflected in the analysis of utility access in other North Carolina ETJs, like those studied in Mebane (2, 3), Pinehurst (9), and the eight

ETJs studies in Parnell et al. (4), the historical causes of this disparity are complex and depend on the unique social context of each town. However, there are some notable spatial patterns within each ETJ that appear to support the trends identified in the regressions.

Utility access

Roanoke Rapids

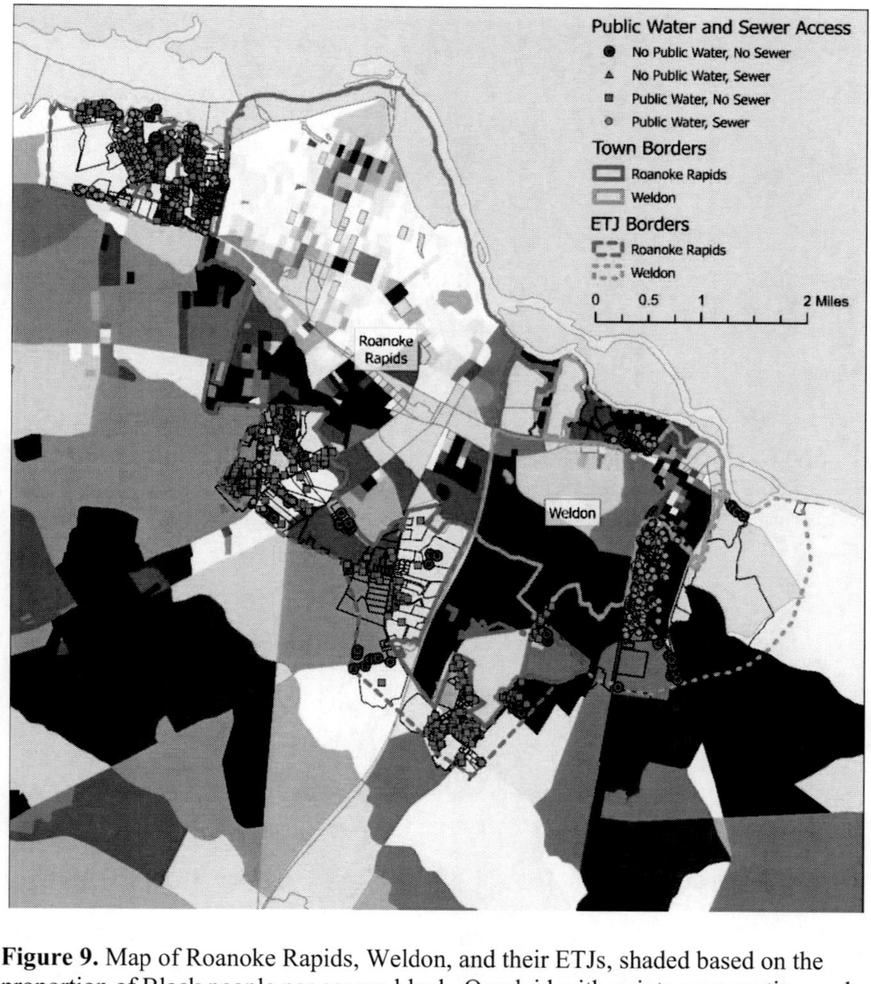

Figure 9. Map of Roanoke Rapids, Weldon, and their ETJs, shaded based on the proportion of Black people per census block. Overlaid with points representing each residence within the ETJs, colored based on their utility access.

In the Roanoke Rapids ETJ (see figure 9), the association between race and utility access appears to be driven by differences between the northern (figure 10a) and southern (figure 10b) sections of the ETJ. These two sections differ greatly in demographics – the mean proportion of Black people per census block is only 0.21 in the northern section, as compared to 0.48 in the southern section and 0.51 in the county overall.

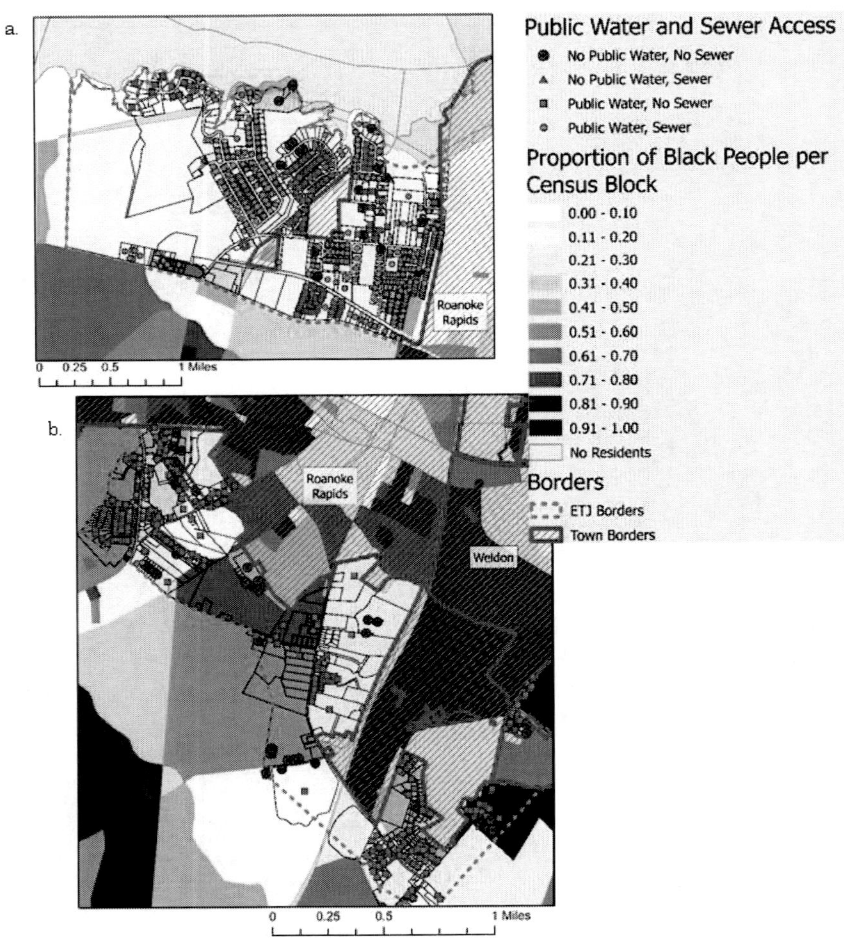

Figure 10. Map of the ETJs of Roanoke Rapids, shaded based on the proportion of Black people per census block. Figure 10a highlights the predominantly white northern section, and 10b highlights the more diverse southern section that has less access to utilities.

In the predominantly white northern section (figure 10a), most residents have access to both public water and sewer (67.1%), with almost all residents having public water (95.2%), and very few lacking both (3.9%), as summarized in Table 4. These observations are reflected in figure 10a, where we see most residences either have both services or have public water without sewer.

Table 4. Comparison of access statistics and demographics between the northern and southern section of the Roanoke Rapids ETJ

	Northern ETJ Section (n = 462)		**Southern ETJ Section (n = 319)**	
	Percent	Count	Percent	Count
Public water only	28.10%	130	74.90%	239
Sewer only	0.90%	4	0%	0
Both public water and sewer	67.10%	310	12.90%	41
Neither public water nor sewer	3.90%	18	12.20%	39
Mean proportion of Black people per census block	0.19		0.48	

However, in the southern section, which has a higher average proportion of Black people per block (0.48), we see less access to both services. Few residents have access to both water and sewer (12.9%), and while a majority still have access to public water, the percentage of access is less than in the northern section (87.8%). Additionally, a greater percentage of residents have neither public water nor sewer (12.2%). This is reflected in figure 10b, where we see both a higher proportion of Black people overall and greater spatial variation in the proportion of Black people.

It was hypothesized that this disparity may be explained by the distance from the WWTP. People who live closer to the plant are expected to be more likely to have access to sewer service than those who live farther away. However, based on the least-cost path between each parcel and the WWTP (figure 11), we found that this is unlikely to be an explanation for the disparity. First, the strong negative correlation (-0.65) between the proportion of Black people per census block and distance from the WWTP suggests that census blocks with a higher proportion of Black people are generally closer to the plant than census blocks with fewer Black residents. When paired with the results of the regression when considering the effect of the relative distance from the plant, which determined that ETJ residents who live farther from the WWTP are more likely to have sewer access than those who live closer (OR: 1.81, $p<0.001$), we see evidence that proximity is not a protective factor for sewer access, as hypothesized. Rather we see that residents who live farther away (i.e., in the northern section), who are also more likely to be white, are more likely to have sewer access than the predominantly Black residents who live closer to the WWTP.

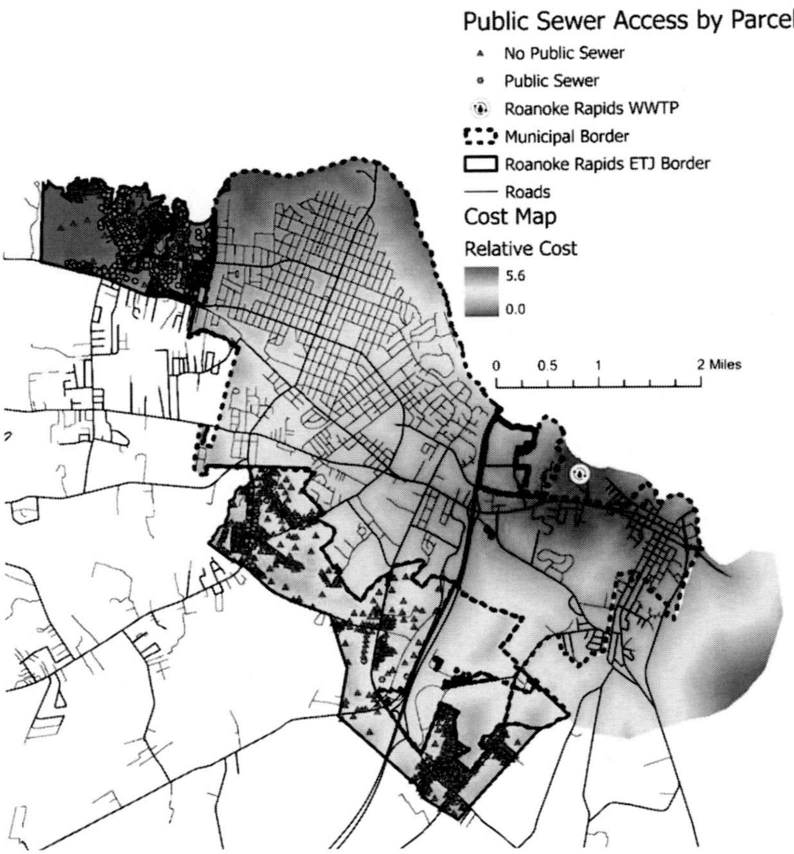

Figure 11. Map highlighting the relative "cost," calculated on the least cost path between a residence and the wastewater treatment plant, and whether or not a residence has sewer service. Most parcels in the northern section of the ETJ have sewer access, but few in the southern section have sewer access.

These observations appear to support the results of the regressions – residents in the areas with a higher proportion of Black people are less likely to have public water and sewer service when accounting for population density, the tax value of the home, and the ownership status of the resident(s).

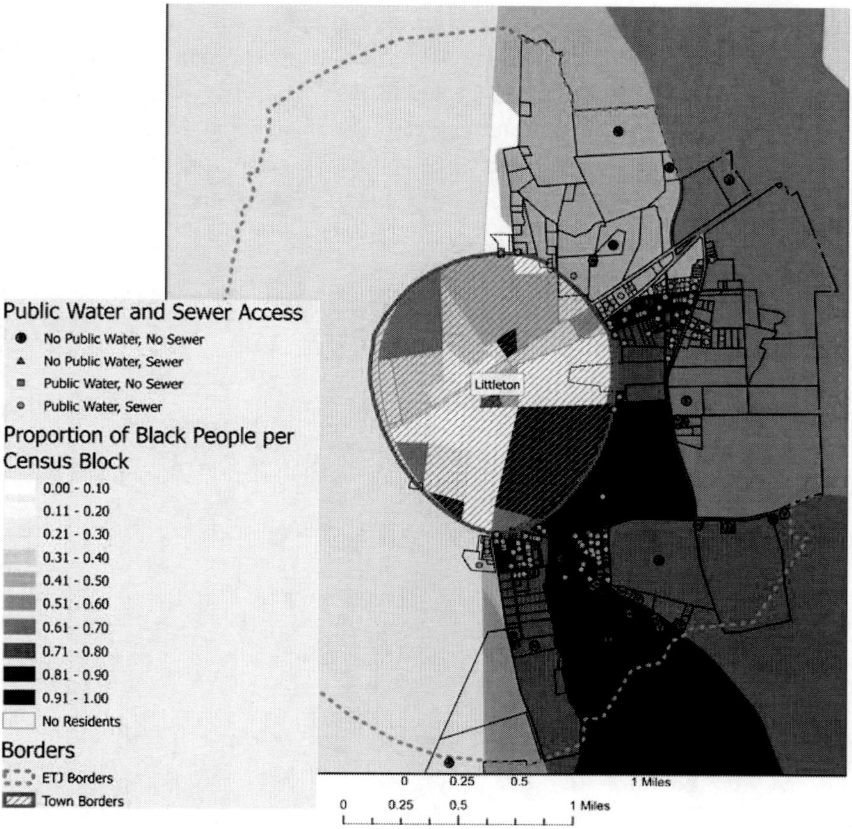

Figure 12. Map of the ETJ of Littleton, shaded based on the proportion of Black people per census block and overlaid with points representing each residence within the ETJs, shaded based on their utility access.

Littleton

In the Littleton ETJ (figure 12), most parcels have access to both public water and sewer (77.4%), and the remaining have neither public water nor sewer access (21.9%) with the exception of a single parcel that has public water service but not sewer service.

Within the ETJ, two residential clusters appear to drive the regression results. One cluster to the south with a high proportion of Black residents, and one to the east, with a greater proportion of white residents. Most of the homes in the ETJ that lack access to public water and sewer are found in and around the predominantly Black southern section. Notably, while the southern cluster has a slightly higher proportion of Black people, it is also much less dense than the eastern cluster, and the effect of population density in the regression appears to be quite strong when compared to the effect in Roanoke Rapids and Littleton. These patterns suggest that the disparity in utility access within the ETJ is likely related to both race and population density. Overall, while a significant relationship was identified between race and utility access, accounting for population density and other factors, the driver of this relationship is less clear than in Roanoke Rapids.

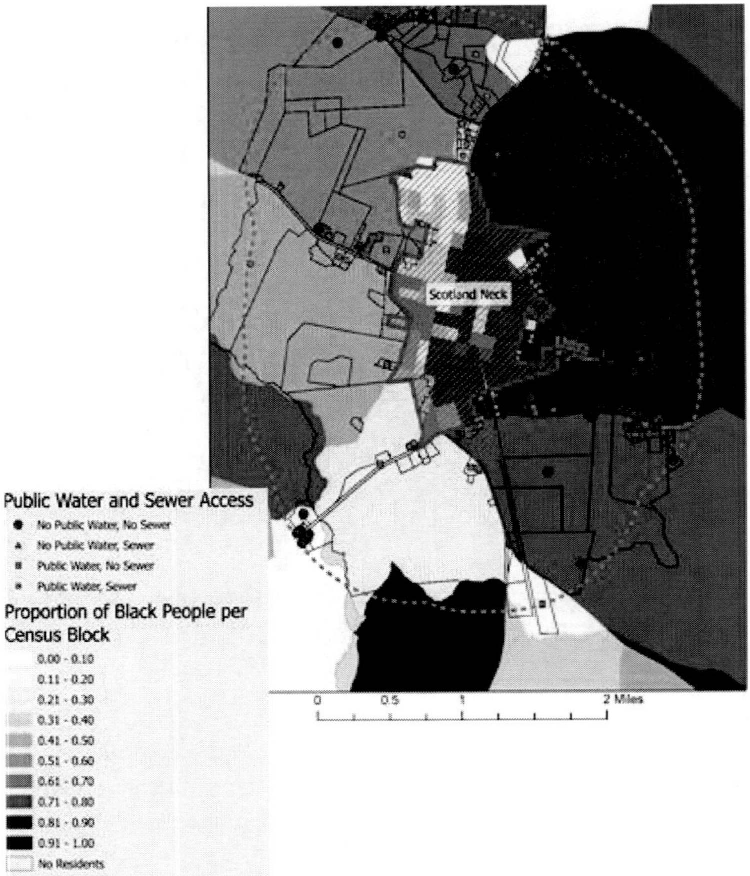

Figure 13. Map of the ETJ of Scotland Neck, shaded based on the proportion of Black people per census block and overlaid with points representing each residence within the ETJs, shaded based on their utility access.

Scotland Neck

In the Scotland Neck ETJ (see figure 13) a significant negative relationship was identified between the proportion of Black people per census block and odds of access to sewer service (OR:0.259, p = 0.032), but not to public water service (p = 0.10). This relationship appears to be driven by the clear divide between the predominantly white region to the west and the predominantly Black region to the east.

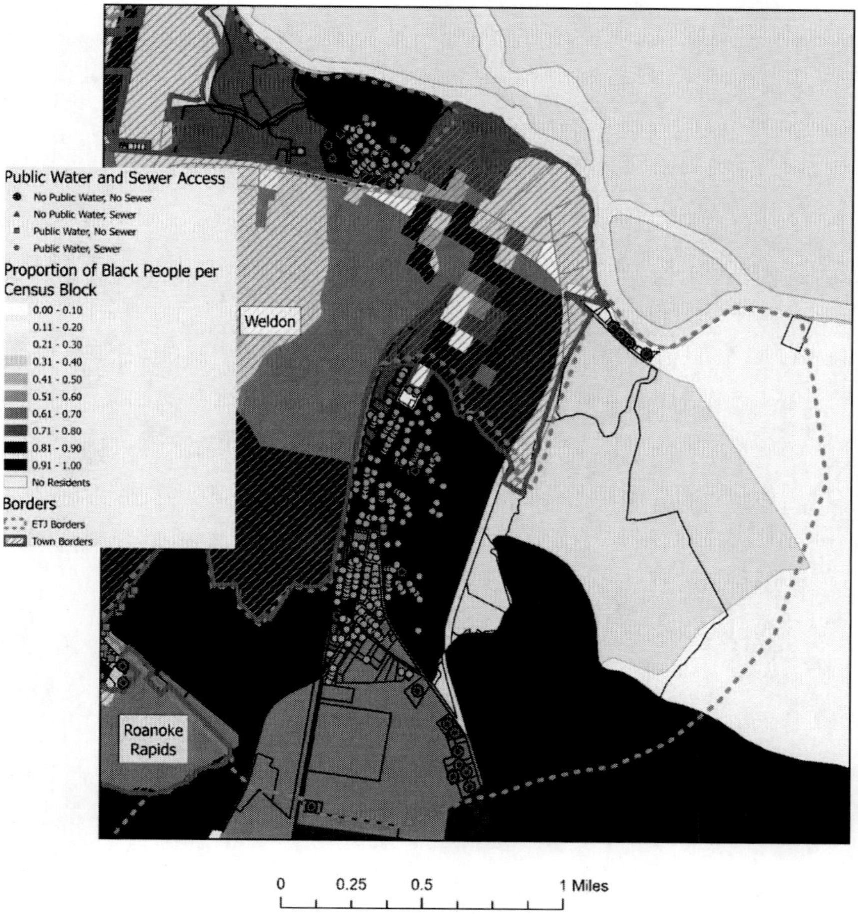

Figure 14. Map of the ETJ of Weldon, shaded based on the proportion of Black people per census block and overlaid with points representing each residence within the ETJs, shaded based on their utility access.

In the predominantly white region, most homes have access to both services with one neighborhood having access to public water but not to sewer and scattered homes lacking access to both. In the predominantly Black eastern section, the only residences with access to sewer are directly bordering the town. When comparing the two regions, in the predominantly white region we see homes almost a mile from the town border with sewer access, yet in the predominantly Black region, where the population density is much higher, we see residences relatively close to the border that do not have sewer access.

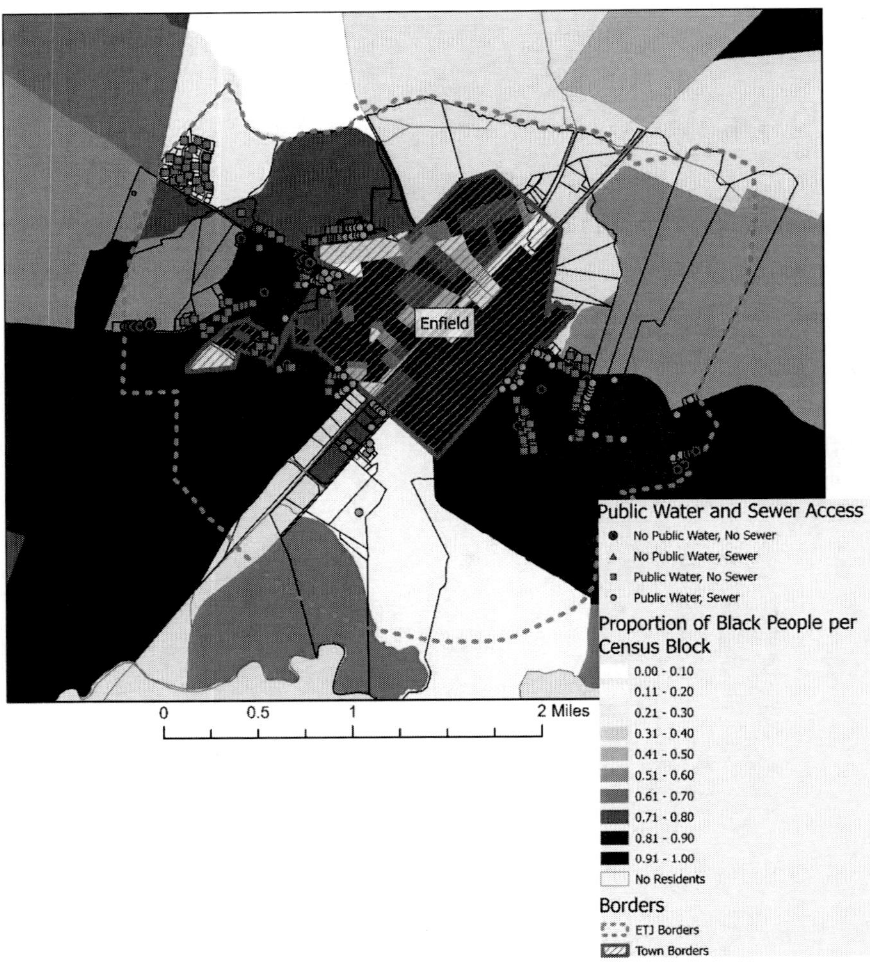

Figure 15. Map of the ETJ of Enfield, shaded based on the proportion of Black people per census block and overlaid with points representing each residence within the ETJs, shaded based on their utility access.

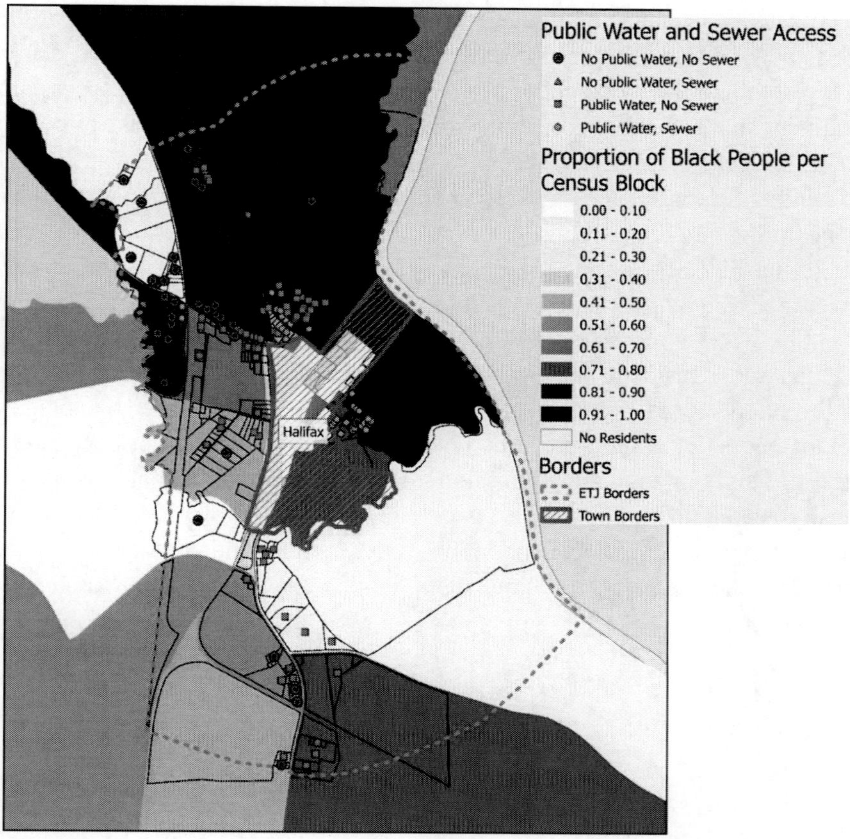

Figure 16. Map of the ETJ of the town of Halifax, shaded based on the proportion of Black people per census block and overlaid with points representing each residence within the ETJs, shaded based on their utility access.

Other ETJs

There does not appear to be a significant relationship between race and access to public utilities in the ETJs of Weldon (figure 14), Enfield (figure 15), and Halifax (figure 16). Potential explanations for this are provided for each town below.

In the Weldon ETJ (figure 14), we believe that the relationship is not statistically significant because almost all residents have access to both public water and sewer, and almost all of the census blocks have a high proportion of Black residents. In other words, a disparity cannot exist because almost every resident has access to both services, and the demographic differences are lesser than those found in other ETJs. In the Enfield ETJ (figure 15), we suspect that there is no statistically significant relationship due to the demographics of the town and ETJ. The residents of Enfield and its ETJ are predominantly Black, so the demographic differences between parcels with and without access are relatively small. Furthermore, almost all ETJ residents have access to public water, so there is no access disparity to begin with, regardless of any racial influences. Similarly, access to sewer appears to follow a pattern of proximity to the border and major roads.

In the ETJ of the town of Halifax (figure 16), it appears that access to sewer is driven by population density (i.e., proximity to the town), and access to public water is unrelated to any variables considered in our analysis. We see that most residents have access to public water – only those on the northwestern edge of the ETJ do not (barring some dispersed residences lacking access). Furthermore, only residents near the town border have sewer access. This supports the regression results, which show that population density is a significant factor in sewer access ($p<0.001$), and that there is no apparent relationship between public water access and any of the other variables. Additionally, the low sample size may have obfuscated any relationships.

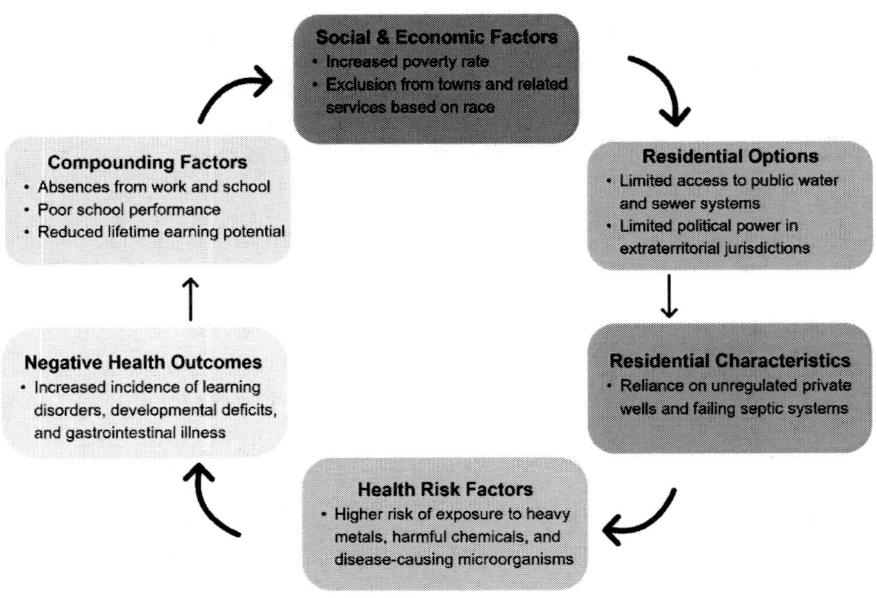

Figure 17. The cycle of environmental health disparities, as manifested in this context.

Cycle of environmental health disparities

The utility access disparities identified in these ETJs and in other underbounded communities can lead to an intergenerational cycle of increased exposure to environmental contaminants (e.g., heavy metals, bacteria, and harmful chemicals) and poorer overall health outcomes (figure 17). Communities that are excluded from public water and sewer services generally utilize private wells and septic systems as alternatives. These systems, which can be difficult and expensive to maintain and repair, are associated with increased exposure to a variety of environmental contaminants. Many contaminants, such as lead and disease-causing microorganisms, can cause negative health outcomes and reduce access to education and employment opportunities.

An example of this cycle is seen in children who are exposed to increased levels of lead in private wells. Lead is a heavy metal and potent neurotoxin that has been found in higher concentrations in private well water when compared to public water (28). Additionally, children who use private wells have been documented as having higher levels of lead in their blood than children who use public water (29). Numerous studies have linked childhood lead exposure with poor academic performance (30), intellectual impairment, and various other developmental deficits that impact overall lifetime earning potential (31).

The use of septic systems is also an important factor in perpetuating the cycle of health disparities. Proximity to a high density of septic systems can lead to an increase in exposure to harmful microorganisms, leading to an increased risk of developing various gastrointestinal illnesses (16). These illnesses can easily lead to expensive emergency department visits, absence from work and school, and other quality-of-life-reducing effects, further limiting earning potential.

These factors can compound and perpetuate a cycle of generational poverty, making it more difficult to address the factors that lead to increased exposure to environmental contaminants. To break this cycle, additional work is needed to identify underbounded communities and provide them with information and support that they can use to advocate for improved services. By working with these underbounded communities and aiding them in securing financial support (e.g., through grants such as Community Development Block Grants through the United States Department of Housing and Urban Development), providing them with legal support, and supporting them in whatever ways they need, researchers, attorneys, and legislators can be an asset for communities that wish to connect to public water and sewer services and improve their health.

Strengths and limitations

The major strength of this study is the use of utility records provided by tax data. In most other studies, public water and sewer access records are not available at a tax parcel level resolution. Instead, access is often estimated in one of two ways. First, based on proximity to service lines (2). This method may overlook parcels that are near service lines but do not have access to services, potentially leading to overestimates in utility access. Or second, based on surveys (3). This method generally limits the scope of the analysis to a smaller area, due to the labor required to conduct accurate large-scale surveys. Due to the presence of utility data in the tax records, we were able to conduct a wide-scale analysis with a level of reliability rarely found in similar studies.

There are several limitations in this study. First, the method for estimating the relative distance from each parcel in the Roanoke Rapids ETJ to the WWTP does not consider the presence of sewer mains running through non-road areas. Therefore, it may overestimate the distance from the WWTP to some parcels. Additionally, we do not consider the effect of time on the distribution of utility pipes. For example, it is possible that the parcels farther from the Roanoke Rapids WWTP are older than the parcels near the WWTP, and thus have had more time to be provided with utilities. Finally, due to the nature of this analysis, it is impossible to draw a causative link between any factors explored in this research and the odds of access to public water and sewer. While we have identified that there is a relationship between the proportion of Black people in a census block and the odds of a parcel having access to public water and sewer in several ETJs, which suggests the presence of bias in the historical apportionment of these services, we cannot claim that this bias is the *cause* of this disparity without more in-depth historical and social research.

Conclusion

Our results show that there is a statistically significant negative association between the proportion of Black people living in a census block and the odds of a residence in that block having access to public water and sewer service in half of the ETJs in Halifax County, North Carolina. In these areas, Black people have been excluded from important public health infrastructure, despite their proximity to said infrastructure, and are therefore more likely to be exposed to factors that adversely impact their well-being and perpetuate a cycle of environmental health disparities.

To better understand the nature of these disparities, additional research focusing on the history and cultural context of each ETJ is necessary. While overt discrimination is less common now than in the past, systemic racism may play a role in the disparities identified here. Systemic racism, the form of racism that is built into the institutional, social, and cognitive structures of a society, can maintain the outcomes of the more overt racism of the past, oftentimes without the intention of harm or even awareness of its existence (32). The effect of systemic racism on the health of marginalized communities, especially Black communities, has been documented in the response to the COVID-19 pandemic (33), policing (34), and almost all institutions in the United States (32). By understanding how systemic racism may manifest in the ETJs of Halifax County, steps can be taken to identify and dismantle the systems that are in place that negatively affect the health of underbounded communities, especially the children of these communities who are most vulnerable

Acknowledgements

We would like to thank Break the Cycle of Health Disparities Inc for its support in the preparation and review of this research. We would also like to thank Riley Mulhern and Michael Fisher for their support in the initial development of this project.

References

[1] Cutler D, Miller G. The role of public health improvements in health advances: The twentieth-century United States. Demography 2005;42(1):1–22.

[2] Johnson JH, Parnell A, Joyner AM, Christman CJ, Marsh B. Racial apartheid in a small North Carolina town. Rev Black Polit Econ 2004;31(4):89–107.

[3] Wilson SM, Heaney CD, Cooper J, Wilson O. Built environment issues in unserved and underserved African-American neighborhoods in North Carolina. Environ Justice 2008;1(2):63–72.

[4] Parnell A, Joyner A, Christman C, Marsh D. The persistence of political segregation: Racial underbounding in North Carolina. Mebane, NC: Cedar Grove Institute Sustainable Communities, 2004.

[5] Purifoy DM. North Carolina [un]incorporated: Place, race, and local environmental inequity. Am Behav Scientist 2021;65(8):1072–103.

[6] Lichter DT, Parisi D, Grice SM, Taquino M. Municipal underbounding: Annexation and racial exclusion in small Southern Towns. 2021;72. URL: http://onlinelibrary.wiley.com/doi/abs/10.1526/003601107781147437.

[7] Aiken CS. Race as a factor in municipal underbounding. Anna Assoc Am Geographers 1987;77(4):564–79.

[8] Shertzer A, Twinam T, Walsh RP. Race, ethnicity, and discriminatory zoning. Am Econ J Appl Economics 2016;8(3):217–46.

[9] Purifoy DM. The plantation town: Race, resources, and the making of place. In: Himley M, Havice E, Valdivia G, eds. The Routledge handbook of critical resource geography, 1st edition. London: Routledge, 2021:114–25.

[10] Local Planning and Development Regulation. G.S. Sect. 160D-202fd. URL: https://www.ncleg.gov/EnactedLegislation/Statutes/PDF/BySection/Chapter_160D/GS_160D-202.pdf.

[11] Owens D. Extraterritorial jurisdiction for planning and development regulation. Chapel Hill, NC: University of North Carolina at Chapel Hill School of Government, 2023. URL: https://www.sog.unc.edu/resources/legal-summaries/extraterritorial-jurisdiction-planning-and-development-regulation.

[12] US Census Bureau. QuickFacts: Halifax County, NC. US Census Bureau, 2020. URL: https://www.census.gov/quickfacts/halifaxcountynorthcarolina.

[13] Parramore T. Tuscarora Indians. In: Powell W, ed. NCpedia. University of North Carolina Press, 2022. URL: https://www.ncpedia.org/american-indians/tuscarora.

[14] Vocci R. Halifax County. NCpedia. Chapel Hill, NC: University of North Carolina Press, 2006. URL: https://www.ncpedia.org/geography/halifax.

[15] US Census Bureau. 1860 Census: Population of the United States. US Census Bureau, 1864. URL: https://www.census.gov/library/publications/1864/dec/1860a.html.

[16] Aiken CS. New settlement pattern of rural blacks in the American south. Geograph Rev 1985;75(4):383–404.

[17] Borchardt MA, Chyou PH, DeVries EO, Belongia EA. Septic system density and infectious diarrhea in a defined population of children. Environ Health Perspect 2003;111(5):742–8.

[18] Stillo F, MacDonald Gibson J. Exposure to contaminated drinking water and health disparities in North Carolina. Am J Public Health 2017;107(1):180–5.

[19] North Carolina Department of Health and Human Services. Private wells: Frequently asked questions about testing. URL: https://epi.dph.ncdhhs.gov/oee/wellwater/faqs.html.

[20] Stillo F, Bruine de Bruin W, Zimmer C, MacDonald Gibson J. Well water testing in African-American communities without municipal infrastructure: Beliefs driving decisions. Sci Total Environ 2019;686:1220–8.

[21] Lanphear BP, Hornung R, Khoury J, Yolton K, Baghurst P, Bellinger DC, et al. Low-level environmental lead exposure and children's intellectual function: An international pooled analysis. Environ Health Perspect 2005;113(7):894–9.

[22] Orange County Health Department. Rogers Road area well and septic survey and assessment report. Orange County Health Department, 2010. URL: https://www.townofchapelhill.org/home/showdocument?id=13077.

[23] Murphy HM, McGinnis S, Blunt R, Stokdyk J, Wu J, Cagle A, et al. Septic systems and rainfall influence human fecal marker and indicator organism occurrence in private wells in Southeastern Pennsylvania. Environ Sci Technol 2020;54(6):3159–68.

[24] Withers PJ, Jordan P, May L, Jarvie HP, Deal NE. Do septic tank systems pose a hidden threat to water quality? Front Ecol Environ 2014;12(2):123–30.

[25] R Core Team. R: A language and environment for statistical computing. Vienna, Austria: R Foundation for Statistical Computing, 2023. URL: https://www.R-project.org/.

[26] RStudio Team. RStudio: Integrated development for R. Boston, MA: RStudio, PBC, 2023. URL: http://www.posit.co/.

[27] Wickham H, Averick M, Bryan J, Chang W, McGowan LD, François R, et al. Welcome to the Tidyverse. J Open Source Software 2019;4(43):1686.

[28] Levin R, Brown MJ, Kashtock ME, Jacobs DE, Whelan EA, Rodman J, et al. Lead exposures in US children, 2008: Implications for prevention. Environ Health Perspect 2008;116(10):1285–93.

[29] MacDonald Gibson J, Fisher M, Clonch A, MacDonald JM, Cook PJ. Children drinking private well water have higher blood lead than those with city water. PNAS 2020;117(29):16898–907.

[30] Miranda ML, Kim D, Galeano MAO, Paul CJ, Hull AP, Morgan SP. The relationship between early childhood blood lead levels and performance on end-of-grade tests. Environ Health Perspect 2007;115(8):1242–7.

[31] Searle AK, Baghurst PA, van Hooff M, Sawyer MG, Sim MR, Galletly C, et al. Tracing the long-term legacy of childhood lead exposure: A review of three decades of the Port Pirie Cohort study. NeuroToxicology 2014;43:46–56.

[32] Banaji MR, Fiske ST, Massey DS. Systemic racism: individuals and interactions, institutions and society. Cogn Res Princ Implic 2021;6:82.

[33] Gravlee CC. Systemic racism, chronic health inequities, and COVID-19: A syndemic in the making? Am J Hum Biol 2020;32(5):e23482.

[34] Richardson R, Schultz J, Crawford K. Dirty data, bad predictions: How civil rights violations impact police data, predictive policing systems, and justice. NYU Law Rev 2019;94:192. URL: https://papers.ssrn.com/abstract=3333423.

Chapter 6

School garden model strategies to combat food insecurity in Lumpkin County, Georgia

Jami Nakan, BS[1,2,*]
Julie Knight-Brown, MS[1]
and David Patterson, PhD[2]
[1]Lumpkin County School District, Lumpkin County, Georgia, United States of America
[2]Department of Biology, The University of North Georgia, Dahlonega, Georgia, United States of America

Food insecurity, as defined by the United States Department of Agriculture, is "a household-level economic and social condition of limited or uncertain access to adequate food." According to the Georgia Department of Education, nearly half of the kindergarten through twelfth-grade students in the Lumpkin County School System in Northeast Georgia are impacted by food insecurity. To address this issue, classes from a local elementary school in Lumpkin County participated in a small-scale garden project designed to provide students with agricultural education and fresh produce from an on-site garden. Classroom evaluations demonstrate that the project was effective in teaching fifth-grade students basic STEM topics centered on garden activities, including botany, physiology, and agricultural practices, while also providing a source of fresh produce. This model offers a simple and effective strategy to address childhood food insecurity and sustainable agricultural education in rural districts in Georgia.

---

* Corresponding Author's E-mails: jnaka9591@ung.edu; jam.nakan@gmail.com

In: Neighborhoods: Impact on Child Health and Development
Editors: I Leslie Rubin and Joav Merrick
ISBN: 979-8-89530-834-9

Introduction

The United States Department of Agriculture defines food insecurity as "a household-level economic and social condition of limited or uncertain access to adequate food" (1). This condition often affects not just a single household but can have intergenerational impacts. Rural communities are disproportionately affected by limited access to fresh produce, compounded by the distances to markets. Feeding America's 2022 report found that nine out of ten counties in the United States with the highest food insecurity rates are classified as rural (2). Consequently, children in rural communities are more likely to experience food insecurity.

Many schools in the United States offer food for students to purchase during school sessions. For poor families struggling with the added cost of school meals, the free and reduced lunch program provides discounted or free meals to qualifying families based on school district and state requirements. The 2022 USDA guidelines for a family of four set the income threshold at $51,338 or less for reduced-price lunch and $36,075 or less for free lunch (3). In 2022, more than 49% of kindergarten through twelfth-grade public school students in Georgia qualified for the free and reduced lunch program (4).

Students are impacted by food insecurity in various ways: (i) financially, they may carry a negative or zero school lunch account balance; (ii) logistically, they may have difficulty obtaining food during school breaks or closures; and (iii) socially and emotionally, they may face judgment from more affluent peers. These challenges can lead to a range of adverse physical, emotional, and social health outcomes. A study on parents' perspectives regarding their child's mental health found that food insecurity in the home is associated with poor child health and development, as well as maternal depression (5). Participants in this study commonly reported experiencing depression, stress, anxiety, and fear (5). Figure 1 illustrates how social and economic stresses contribute to food insecurity and related health disparities.

In this context, addressing the challenge of food insecurity in rural elementary schools and breaking the cycle of consequential health disparities, requires the provision of affordable and nutritional food that is also available during school closures, as well as providing educational opportunities that facilitate small-scale gardening at school and/or within homes of the children and their families, to promote sustainability. This model offers a possible solution to the persistent and growing problem of childhood food insecurity through small-scale, community gardens accompanied by nutritional and agricultural education, that is integrated into rural school systems. In addition, a school-based, small-scale educational community garden could help to address disparities in mental and physical health by providing opportunity for outdoor productive physical activity affording the green space for stress relief (6, 7), at the same time as reducing food security through access to fresh produce. School-based community gardens could also function as a way for families to gather fresh produce, particularly in settings where there may be difficulty implementing a formalized charity fruit and vegetable distribution system, or where there is a social stigma associated with the need for food assistance and food access.

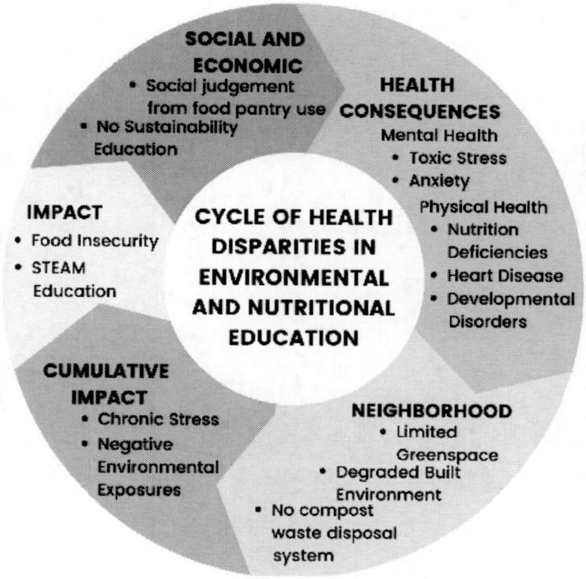

Figure 1. Cycle diagram.

We, therefore, proposed the establishment of an Elementary School Garden Model program for elementary school-aged children by implementing environmental and nutritional education, and providing sustainable produce for students to break the cycle of food insecurity. This program will help to address the immediate needs of hunger and food insecurity, while also educating students about healthy eating and sustainable community gardening, thereby providing not only immediate relief for food insecurity, but also provide a foundation for good nutritional health and a measure of self-sufficiency after graduating from the K-12 system.

This project centered on developing a school-based garden model to provide hands-on education projects for students that can be fully integrated into the existing school curriculum. This initiative reflected current school standards while furthering an understanding of many important scientific topics, such as Science, Technology, Engineering, Art, and Math (STEAM), a popular and effective education focus in school systems. Community gardens can be integrated into a well-rounded STEAM education and can lead to an expanded set of career opportunities. For example, learning about growing plants which may appeal to students who are interested in garden design, composting, soil science, nutrition and health, and environmental education or could inspire some children to pursue career paths that may lead to farming or landscaping, or into research in agriculture, environmental sciences, and engineering.

This project explored the implementation and impact of a school garden program on the educational experiences of second and fifth graders in the Lumpkin County School System in Georgia, USA in agricultural and nutritional domains, while also providing access to nutritious produce thus reducing food insecurity.

We aimed to answer whether a two-pronged project involving the scientific study of gardening and small-scale agriculture production can (a) serve as an educational vehicle for learning botany, practicing sustainability, and exposing students to agricultural skills and careers, and (b) serve as a means of introducing alternative sources of food access, through locally grown healthy fruits and vegetables to reduce food insecurity.

Our study

A school-based community garden project was implemented through Hometown Harvest, a university garden run by student and faculty volunteers as a part of The University of North Georgia (UNG) located in Lumpkin County, GA, United States. Hometown Harvest focuses on growing a variety of fruits and vegetables dictated by the needs of the school system, which include okra, carrots and muscadines, are donated to the local K-12 school system in Lumpkin County. Funding for the project was provided by The University of North Georgia STEM Grant and Biology Department, and the Whole Kids Foundation.

Precision agriculture technology

One of the challenges of every growing season is adapting to the ever-changing environmental conditions of Appalachia. Precision agriculture technology (PAT) is a device employed to measure soil moisture and temperature conditions, using probes placed in the soil. PAT soil moisture probes send out small electric signals into the soil, then use a resistor to measure moisture according to the amount of electricity received. The standard rule is that damp soil will have less resistance than dry soil, resulting in data that reflects moisture levels measured in centibars.

To begin this project, multiple garden locations around the Hometown Harvest garden were tested to find the best agricultural and moisture conditions for growing spring and summer plants, specifically collard greens. Collard green seeds were planted and tested over two garden seasons, to determine if dramatic temperature and moisture fluctuations would cause stress in the plants (8).

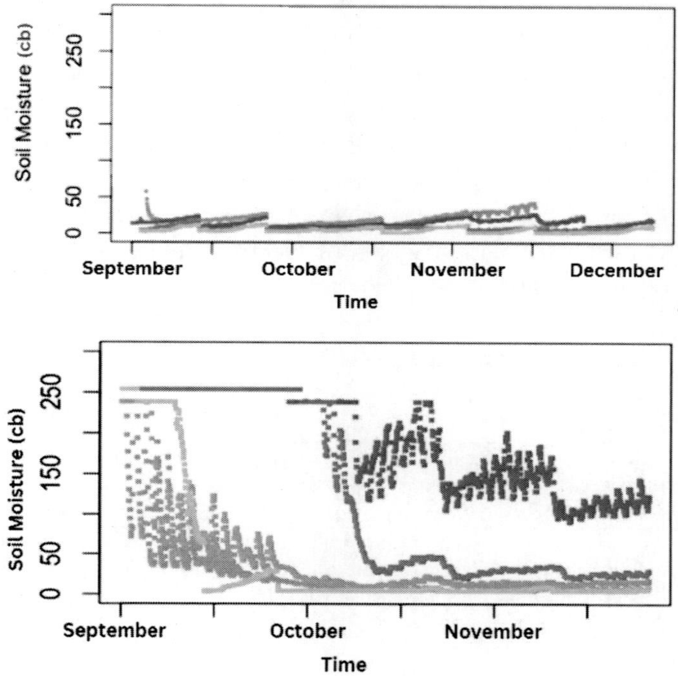

a.

b.

Figure 2. Each line represents the effects of soil moisture levels on a variety of plants during winter 2022.

Preliminary results found that overwatered plants have a larger yield but poorer quality produce. The PAT system produced two graphs via R. One graph explored high, yet varying, levels of moisture (see figure 2b), while another assessed very low levels of moisture that peaked at around 50 centibars (see Figure 2a). Using these data, we observed that the pilot garden did not require frequent watering or maintenance to function in a north Georgia school, requiring only a 50 centibar moisture condition, demonstrating that the garden received very little water during the winter season, yet collard greens grew successfully. Thus, soil conditions reflecting these moisture conditions ultimately leads to a higher yield, which results in an increased amount of produce available to students in the school system.

Assessing educational model outcomes

To test a new curriculum model, we collaborated with a local elementary school in Lumpkin County to determine if a school-based community garden would help students learn about topics in three major categories: agriculture, sustainability, and botany. Lumpkin County Public Schools follow guidelines from the state government called the Georgia Standards of Excellence. Current K-5 Georgia education standards were reviewed for the purpose of creating a framework to assess educational outcomes. Identified education standards applicable to the garden project are listed in the table below (see table 1) (9-11). The pilot garden curriculum was shaped to meet these learning standards in conjunction with the current goals of Georgia Public Schools and the Lumpkin County School Nutrition Program.

Table 1. Georgia State K-12 Standards (9, 10, 11)

Standard	Objective
S5L1.c	Develop a model that illustrates how plants are sorted into groups (seed producers, non-seed producers) using data from multiple sources
HE2.1.e:	Identify proper nutrition that provides energy to help the body grow and develop
S3L1.:	Obtain, evaluate, and communicate information about the similarities and differences between plants, animals, and habitats found within geographic regions (Blue Ridge Mountains, Piedmont, Coastal Plains, Valley and Ridge, and Appalachian Plateau) of Georgia

To assess educational outcomes, a pre-course test (Pre-Test) was administered in both second grade (n = 19) and fifth grade (n = 67) classes.

The second-grade exam involved reading each question aloud in a classroom setting and answering any clarification questions on word definitions. The fifth-grade exam was administered in writing, using a silent classroom setting. All exams were in person and the questions were presented on paper.

Exams were administered for twenty minutes. During this time both teachers and administrative staff were present, as well as the research team to proctor. This Pretest exam was made up of six questions for the second graders and seven questions for the fifth graders. Each major topic included two questions, designed to overlap with concepts suggested by the school nutrition staff. Exams primarily featured multiple choice-style questions, but also involved a timeline question (as students were asked to place garden processes in order of events), and a section for matching proper compost materials to a compost container.

Because a 2020 study concluded that students tend to prefer multiple-choice style questions in an academic environment but did not find a significant difference between using multiple-choice questions and open-ended questions (12), we structured our test in accordance with their suggestions and featured multiple choice questions as well as matching questions. The project relied on a foundation built by current K-12 Georgia Standards concepts, so a unique test design was achieved through colorful images and words as well as the opportunity to receive assistance with question comprehension from the exam administrator (see Table 3 and 4). Students were assured by classroom instructors that the results of the exams would not impact their grades or recorded academic performance.

After the pre-test, we partnered with classroom teachers to conduct a 5-day educational classroom and hands-on garden course for the second and fifth grade students. Students participated in a variety of activities geared toward the learning objective. The details of the 5-day program are listed below (see Table 2).

Based on our experience from our Hometown Harvest garden, radishes were chosen to be the vegetable of focus because of their fast growth time, nutritional value, and their tolerance of early spring conditions. Collard greens and tomatoes were considered for the project but were ultimately rejected due to planting time and size respectively. While collard greens were the focus of prior studies within Hometown Harvest, radishes were chosen for study in the elementary school garden curriculum proposal, because while collard greens are typically grown in the winter months, radishes are relatively smaller plants that can be grown easily in planter boxes and grow well during the Spring Semester (January-May).

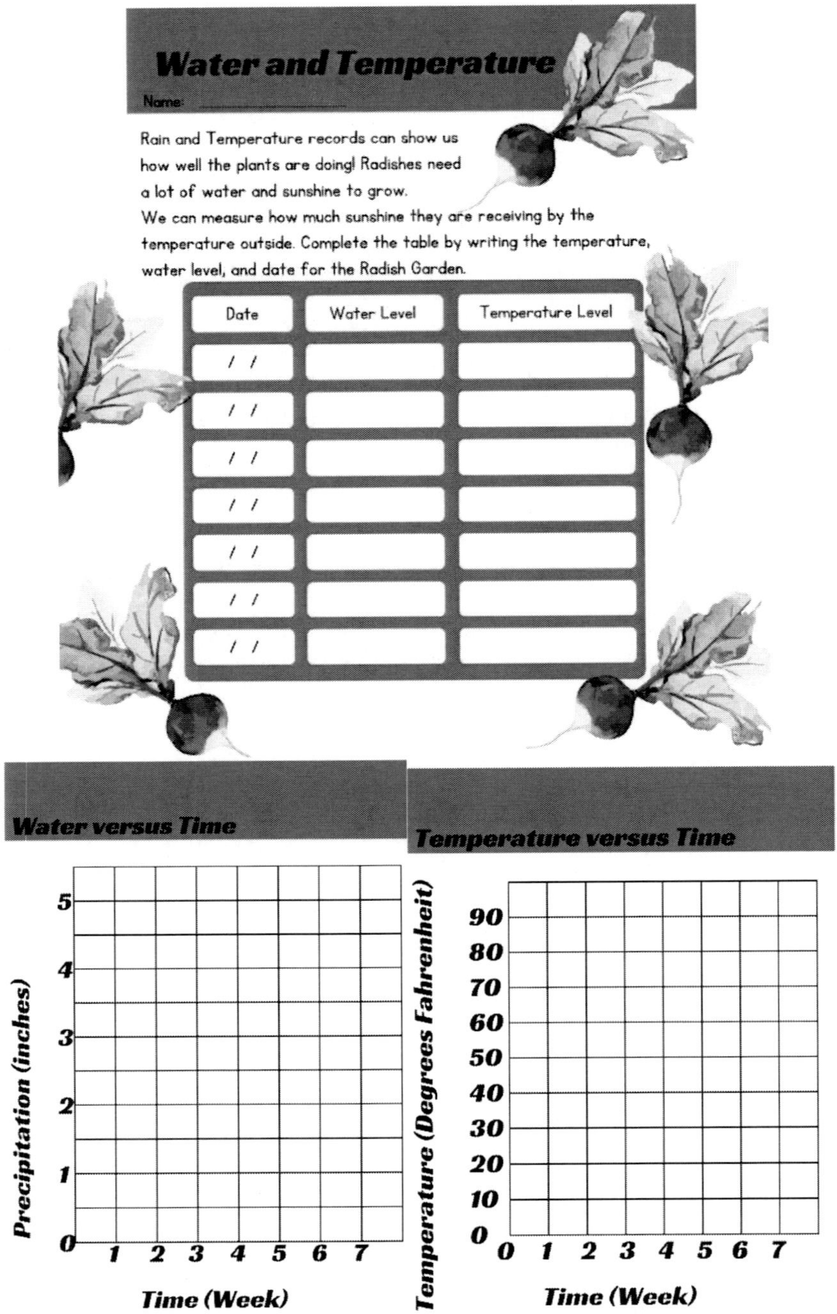

Water and Temperature

Name: ____________

Rain and Temperature records can show us how well the plants are doing! Radishes need a lot of water and sunshine to grow.
We can measure how much sunshine they are receiving by the temperature outside. Complete the table by writing the temperature, water level, and date for the Radish Garden.

Date	Water Level	Temperature Level
/ /		
/ /		
/ /		
/ /		
/ /		
/ /		
/ /		

Figure 3. Garden data record worksheets.

Teachers randomly assigned students into groups of four or five to conduct the experiment. Each group maintained their own planter box, sustainably made from 100% recycled plastic, and sourced from a local hardware store. Each planter box was of the same dimension and labeled with a number representing each group.

Radish seeds were sown in February 2023 with the aim of a harvest by the end of the school semester in May. Instead of being instructed specifically on PAT, students monitored the temperature via an analog outdoor thermometer and measured water levels using a glass rain gauge, for cost-efficiency purposes. Each fifth-grade group was given the task of working together to maintain a graph and chart data points (temperature and water levels) which were collected weekly for about 9 weeks (see Figure 3). The second graders were given the task of working together as a class to plot water and temperature data points and were given extra assistance in finding the data points (as they had not yet been taught the application of measurement systems like assessing temperature and rainfall levels).

Each classroom session in the program began with a pre-test, followed by collecting garden data and completing worksheets on topics such as botany or sustainability, ending with a classroom discussion of the real-life application of the learning goals.

Table 2. Classroom activity and topic schedule by grade level

	Grade Level	
	Second Grade	Fifth Grade
Course Day 1 Learning Topic: Botany	- Pre-Test - Basic Botany Lesson with Plant Organ Identification	- Pre-Test - Advanced Botany Lesson with Plant Organ Identification - PAT Preview
Course Day 2 Learning Topic: Agriculture	- Garden Construction Day with Seed Sowing - Water and Temperature Data Collection Chart Setup	- Garden Construction Day with Seed Sowing - Water and Temperature Data Collection Chart Setup
Course Day 3 Learning Topic: Agriculture	- Garden Maintenance - Water and Temperature Data Collection Check-In	- Garden Maintenance - Water and Temperature Data Collection Check-In
Course Day 4 Learning Topic: Sustainability	- Composting Lesson and Worksheet - Water and Temperature Data Collection Check-In	- Composting Lesson and Worksheet - Water and Temperature Data Collection Check-In
Course Day 5	- Post-Test - Water and Temperature Data Collection Check-In	- Post-Test - Water and Temperature Data Collection Check-In

The topic for day one of instruction focused on basic botany (e.g., labeling a seed, identifying common plants, and learning how to take care of a growing plant) for both the second and fifth graders. Students were encouraged to discuss their experience with plants with others; the fifth-grade class received a preview of PAT and learned what a graph from a machine may look like (see figure 2). The second-grade class learned about garden setup and discussed agriculture; the fifth-grade class focused on learning about different classifications of plants, such as Vascular and Nonvascular (13). The third day of class involved garden maintenance for all classes. This included watering the plants and growth observation. The fourth day of class focused on composting and the fifth day of class involved administering the post-test. The post-test was identical to the pre-test in both content and administration, to determine how class knowledge improved throughout participation in the program. Table 2 below organizes the activities into a 5-day schedule of topics (see table 2).

We hypothesized that all fifth and second grade classes would increase their scores from the pre-test to the post-test in all categories after our five-day curriculum. We also expected students to have a working knowledge of basic gardening techniques by the end of the course.

Findings

The fifth grade and second grade classroom data were graded and analyzed separately. Four students were absent during the Post-Test in the fifth-grade class, resulting in only 63 of the 67 students participating. Scores are presented through a percentage format to reflect the change. Fifth-grade students were subdivided into three classrooms: Class 1, Class 2, and Class 3. These classes have a combined average score increase of 18.11% (see figure 4). This score scale used partial credit for overall concept knowledge, as questions often carried discrete prompts inside. These prompts include questions that assess knowledge of more than one topic within the subject categories.

Tables 3 and 4 display each question on the exam organized by subject category (Sustainability, Agriculture, and Botany) for fifth and second grade levels. A breakdown of each question without partial credit is displayed below for the fifth grade (see table 3).

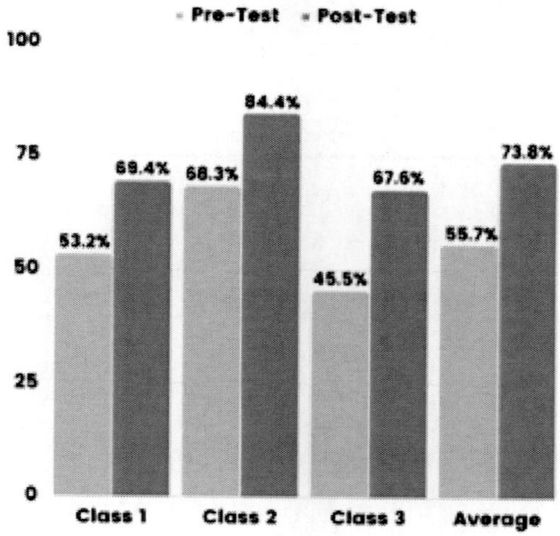

Figure 4. Fifth grade exam performance.

Table 3. Number of fifth grade students who answered full question correctly (no partial credit)

	Pre-Course Test	**Post-Course Test**
	n (5th Grade): 67	n (5th Grade): 63
Soil Conditions (Agriculture)	Question: Which plant graph produced the best quality vegetables? Possible Answers: (a. 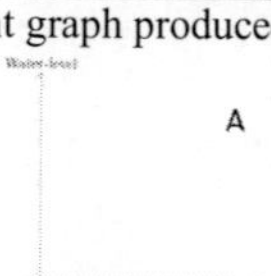 b. 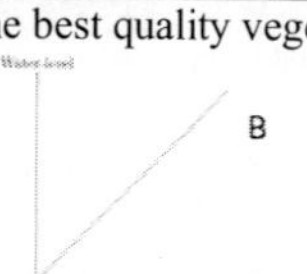 c. 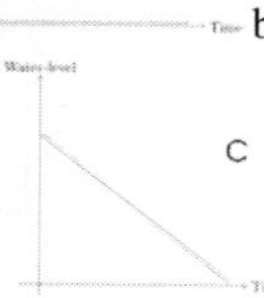 d. 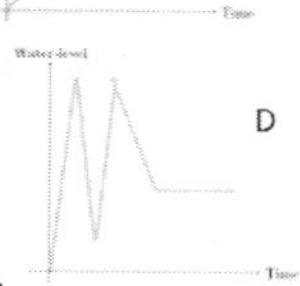) Correct Answer: B	
Percentage of Students with Correct Answer	38.81%	49.25%
Garden Timeline (Agriculture)	Question: Put the following steps in order using the letters on the lines below. Possible Answers: (a. Prepare the Soil With Compost, b. Compost scraps for the next garden, c. Examine Quality and Quantity, d. Harvest, e. Water and Monitor Water Levels, f. Sow Seeds) Correct Answer: A, F, E, D, C, B	

Table 3. (Continued)

	Pre-Course Test	Post-Course Test
	n (5th Grade): 67	n (5th Grade): 63
Percentage of Students with Correct Answer	7.46%	7.46%
Compost (Sustainability)	Question: Circle all of the following that can go into a compost pile: Possible Answers: (a. Banana, b. Apple, c. Soda Can, d. Carrot, e. Cheese, f. Grass, g. Glass, h. Bacon, i. Ice Cream, j. Paper) Correct Answer: A, B, D, F, J	
Percentage of Students with Correct Answer	5.97%	73.13%
True or False (Nutrition and Sustainability)	Question I. Radishes are less healthy than pizza Question II. Radishes give you vitamins and minerals Question III. They help to take away air pollution Question IV. Radish plants take away oxygen Question V. They keep your heart healthy Question VI. Radishes keep your lungs unhealthy Possible Answers: (True or False) Correct Answers: I False, II True, III True, IV False, V	
Percentage of Students with Correct Answer	4.48%	14.93%
Plant Systems (Botany)	Question: What is a vascular plant? Possible Answers: (a. Plants that have tubes to transport water and food, b. Plants that have tubes to transport water and air, c. Plants that don't have tubes) Correct Answer: A	
Percentage of Students with Correct Answer	52.24%	76.12%
Plant Systems (Botany)	Question: What is a non-vascular plant? Possible Answers: (a. A large plant that lacks true roots, stems, and leaves, b. A small plant that lacks true roots, stems, and leaves, c. A small plant that has true roots, stems, and leaves, d. A large plant that has true roots, stems, and leaves.) Correct Answer: B	
Percentage of Students with Correct Answer	50.75%	77.61%
Plant Systems (Botany)	Question: What is an example of a non-vascular plant? Possible Answers: (a. Moss, b. Pine Tree, c. Radish) Correct Answer: A	
Percentage of Students with Correct Answer	65.67%	88.06%

The average score for each fifth-grade subject category improved. In Botany concepts, the average score increased by 28.7%. In Agriculture, the average score increased by 9.7%. Sustainability scores increased by 11.5%.

The second-grade students demonstrated very different results (see table 4). Although Agriculture scores rose by 8.3%, Sustainability dropped by 1.3% and Botany lowered by 3.3%.

Table 4. Number of second grade students who answered full question correctly (no partial credit)

	Pre-Course Test	Post-Course Test
	n (2nd Grade): 19	n (2nd Grade): 19
Soil Conditions (Agriculture)	Question: Which plant graph produced the best quality vegetables? Possible Answers: (a. b. c. d.) 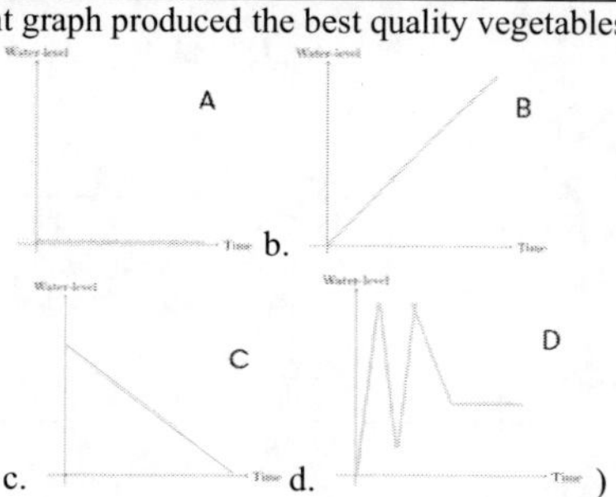 Correct: B	
Percentage of Students with Correct Answer	36.84%	47.37%
Garden Timeline (Agriculture)	Question: Put the following steps in order using the letters on the lines below. Possible Answers: (. Prepare the Soil With Compost, b. Compost scraps for the next garden, c. Count good-looking radishes, d. Harvest, e. Water and Look at Water Levels, f. Sow Seeds) Correct Answers: A, F, E, D, C, B	
Percentage of Students with Correct Answer	5.26%	0%
Compost (Sustainability)	Question: Circle all of the following that can go into a compost pile: Possible Answers: (a. Banana, b. Apple, c. Soda Can, d. Carrot, e. Cheese, f. Grass, g. Glass, h. Bacon, i. Ice Cream, j. Paper) Correct Answers: A, B, D, F, J	
Percentage of Students with Correct Answer	0%	26.32%
True or False (Nutrition and Sustainability)	Question I. Radishes are less healthy than pizza Question II. Radishes give you vitamins and minerals Question III. They help to take away air pollution Question IV. Radish plants take away oxygen Question V. They keep your heart healthy Question VI. Radishes keep your lungs unhealthy Possible Answers: (True or False) Correct Answers: I False, II True, III True, IV False, V	

Table 4. (Continued)

	Pre-Course Test	Post-Course Test
	n (2nd Grade): 19	n (2nd Grade): 19
Percentage of Students with Correct Answer	10.53%	0%
Plant Sstems (Botany)	Question: What do plant roots do? Possible Answers: (a. Roots flower, b. Roots hold energy and flower, c. Roots hold energy and take up water and soil minerals, d. Roots can grow leaves with sunshine and water) Correct Answer: C	
Percentage of Students with Correct Answer	47.37%	36.84%
Plant Systems (Botany)	Question: What do plants need to grow? Possible Answers: (a. Seed + Water + Sun + Compost + Time, b. Seed + Water + Sun + Soil + Groundhogs, c. Seed + Water + Sun + Time + Plastic Container) Correct Answer: A	
Percentage of Students with Correct Answer	73.68%	84.21%

Overall, the average second grade score decreased by 0.66% which was not statistically significant. The pre-test average for the second-grade class was 47.80%. The post-test average score was 47.14%.

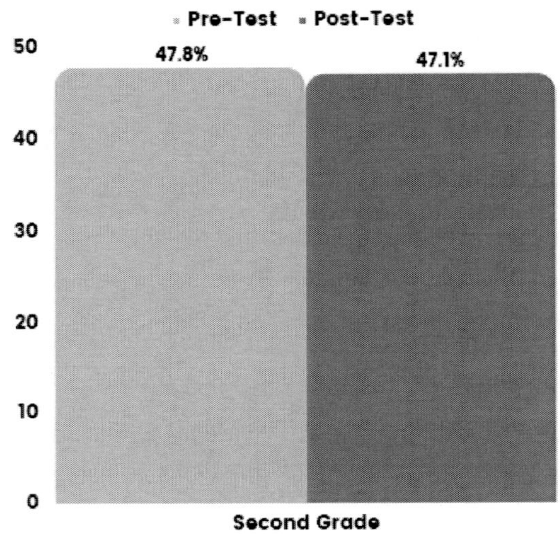

Figure 5. Second grade exam performance.

Discussion

Recognizing the high rate of food insecurity among school children in rural North Georgia and the adverse impact of food insecurity on health, development, and learning, we developed a small scale school community garden with the aim of learning whether involving the elementary school students in the process, (i) could serve as an educational opportunity for learning botany, practicing sustainability, and exposing students to agricultural skills and careers, at the same time as (ii) reducing food insecurity, through locally grown healthy fruits and vegetables. We chose to test this hypothesis on second- and fifth-graders in the school. Results of the pre- and post-test scores for the fifth-grade students confirmed our hypothesis that school garden programs benefit elementary school students academically, as student knowledge of identified educational standards improved by the end of the course. We predicted that school garden models would help students' understanding of basic botany and sustainability and potentially provide a future source of produce for the school.

Our finding of an overall decrease in scores for second-grade students was puzzling and suggests a possible error with either with the course development and/or aspects of the administration or the language of the tests. Some language was adapted from the fifth-grade exam in an attempt to meet the written reading level of second-graders according to Georgia Standards of Excellence (9, 10), but did not account for gaps in learning; possibly, in part, because of the coincidental timing of the COVID-19 Pandemic, or the limited experience of the author of the test. A proposed improvement is to include images representing the words on the exam, and graphics in the administered curricular materials to facilitate understanding and engagement. In the future, it may be beneficial to have elementary-level science classroom teachers review the exams and assignments before presenting them to students. Of note, second grade students did subjectively express satisfaction with the curriculum.

Furthermore, classroom discussions provided robust insights into the most beneficial parts of this education project through comments, reflections, and conversations. Students from both the second and fifth grades spoke about their own experiences with agriculture. Qualitative analysis could potentially yield valuable information, as taking the time to listen to the students speak about their perspectives contributed significantly to the project. The listening process allowed the students express their hopes for the future and enabled learners of all ages to connect to their peers and teachers, thereby forming collaborations that will be beneficial on their future educational journeys.

Strengths and limitations

Overall, this project supports the inclusion of education strategies centered around promoting experiential learning in a positive and productively active outdoor environment while addressing food insecurity in the context of the cycle of health disparities (see figure 1) (16). The positive impact on fifth-grade students in learning about the process and benefits of participating in the establishment of a community garden is reflected in their satisfaction with the curriculum and classroom activities. Anecdotally, the fifth-grade teachers noted that, upon completing the garden program, their students felt more prepared for their biology exams.

A limitation of this project is that the measured outcomes for the second-grade students was not consistent with expectations and requires a critical review and revision of the teaching and testing materials. Another significant limitation was in the time constraint, which dictated what we could plant and what we could do, for example, we would have liked to implement a school compost bin in the cafeteria to further engage the students in hands-on learning about recycling and its role in soil enrichment, thus proving them with a connection between the growing and the eating and the positive value use of food waste.

Conclusion

In summary, we found that introduction of educational innovations to existing curricula in school systems by incorporating and maintaining school-based community gardens, could provide a positive learning experience for the children around the process of growing food and, at the same time, serve to reduce food insecurity among vulnerable children. At a practical level, radish or winter vegetable gardens provide a low maintenance source of organic produce for students while also complimenting the school curriculum due to their application within and expansion upon current educational guidelines. The outcome is that the students have had new experiences that they can build on for their futures, and that with the consumption of the fresh produce will improve their nutrition and overall health.

Based on challenges and successes from our examination process future research should incorporate a qualitative study to determine whether this program is beneficial for students' and/or teachers' educational experiences and mental health. Additionally, any constructive feedback may assist in shaping the program for future applications.

Furthermore, schools could expand libraries to include community gardening literature, as this pilot garden program is a natural launching pad for future learning. A recommended agricultural book series for elementary schools is the Foxfire Books (14), a series that are written records of generations of gardeners and farmers in the southern Appalachia Region.

Although we were not able to install a compost bin during our project period, we recommend the use of a compost bin in any school lunchroom setting, with education on appropriate use. We suggest that senior students participate in educating their younger peers on proper composting techniques and environmental health may assist learning, environmental stewardship, and mentorship. Composting would teach sustainability in tangible ways, by providing an alternative disposal source of food waste and a cost-effective route to replenish soil nutrients (15). In many projects, sustainability practices can lower costs by encouraging the reuse of glass and plastic as garden containers and equipment. We urge school systems globally to construct academic, service-based gardens to empower students to sow the seeds of a brighter future in science and reduce food security and promote sustainability.

Acknowledgments

Disclosure statements: The authors have no financial relationships relevant to this article to disclose. The authors have no conflicts of interest to disclose. The preparation for this project and manuscript review was supported by the Break the Cycle of Health Disparities Program of the Southeast PEHSU at Emory University and Break the Cycle of Health Disparities, Inc. The materials and supplies for the school project were funded and donated by The University of North Georgia STEM Lab, Biology Department, and Hometown Harvest. All of the supplies and funding were donated to the Lumpkin County School System in full for this project. Special thanks to teachers and Lumpkin County School staff for assisting with this project.

References

[1] USDA. Definitions of food security. United States Department of Agriculture Economic Research Service, 2023. URL: https://www.ers.usda.gov/topics/food-nutrition-assistance/food-security-in-the-u-s/definitions-of-food-security/.

[2] Hake M, Engelhard E, Dewey A. Map the Meal Gap 2022, Feeding America 2022:1–8. URL: https://www.feedingamerica.org/sites/default/files/2022-08/Map%20the%20Meal%20Gap%202022%20Report.pdf.

[3] United States Department of Agriculture Food and Nutrition Service Child Nutrition Programs: Income eligibility guidelines. Alexandria, VA: USDA, 2022.

[4] Georgia Department of Education. Free and reduced lunch (FRL) - Fiscal year 2023 Data Report. Free and Reduced Price Meal Eligibility 2023. URL: https://oraapp.doe.k12.ga.us/ows-bin/owa/fte_pack_frl001_public.entry_form.

[5] Knowles MR, Rabinowich J, Ettinger de Cuba S, Cutts DB, Chilton M. "Do you wanna breathe or eat?": Parent perspectives on child health consequences of food insecurity, trade-offs, and toxic stress. Matern Child Health J 2016;20(1):25–32.

[6] de la Osa N, Pastor JBN, Penelo E. Long-term exposure to greenspace and anxiety from preschool and primary school children. J Environ Psychol 2023;93(12): 102207.

[7] Madzia J, Ryan P, Yolton K, Percy Z, Newman N, LeMasters G, et al. Residential greenspace association with childhood behavioral outcomes. J Pediatr 2019;207:233-40.

[8] Mate MD, Zima IS. Development and yield of field tomato under different water supply. Res J Agricultural Sci 2020;52(1):167–77.

[9] Georgia Department of Education. Science Georgia Standards of Excellence: Second-Grade Science Standards 2016. URL: https://lor2.gadoe.org/gadoe/file/60491314-8e51-4220-b4a6-1e55132404fd/1/Science-Second-Grade-Georgia-Standards.pdf.

[10] Georgia Department of Education. Science Georgia Standards of Excellence Fifth-Grade Science Standards 2016. URL: https://www.georgiastandards.org/Georgia-Standards/Documents/Science-Fifth-Grade-Georgia-Standards.pdf.

[11] Georgia Department of Education. Science Georgia Standards of Excellence: Third Grade Science Standards 2016. URL: https://www.georgiastandards.org/Georgia-Standards/Documents/Science-Third-Grade-Georgia-Standards.pdf.

[12] Turhan NS. Why do students prefer different question types? Int J Progr Educ 2020;16(3):132–41.

[13] Georgia Department of Education, Woods R. Georgia Standards of Excellence (GSE). Kindergarten-Grade 5 2021. URL: https://www.georgiastandards.org/Georgia-Standards/Documents/Health-Education-K-5-Georgia-Standards.pdf.

[14] Eliot W, Bennett M. Foxfire. Garden City, NY: Anchor Press/Doubleday, 1984.

[15] Schumpert K, Dietz C, Cycle E. School compost programs: Pathways to success 2012. URL: http://eeingeorgia.org/Files/EE/2012/School_Compost_Programs.pdf.

[16] Break the Cycle of Health Disparities: Atlanta, GA: Break the Cycle. URL: https://www.breakthecycleprogram.org/

Chapter 7

Presence of stressors surrounding local elementary schools in redlined and non-redlined communities in Albany, New York, November–December 2022

**Kaylee Stewart*
and Stacy M Pettigrew†, BA, MS, PhD**
Albany College of Pharmacy and Health Sciences, Albany,
New York, United States of America

Lending patterns based on the 1933 Home Owners' Loan Corporation map characterizations resulted in long lasting and persistent economic and racial disparities. Many neighborhoods deemed 'hazardous' at the time remain low-income today. Poverty can increase children's stress levels, which can result in adverse health effects from childhood into adulthood. Our objective was to determine differences in the presence of stressors surrounding redlined and non-redlined schools in Albany, New York. Data collection consisted of two components: (i) an observational study that evaluated the non-permanent stressors that the students were exposed to and (ii) a mapping identification to locate and evaluate stressors that students were seeing on a regular basis. The Kruskal Wallis one-way analysis of variance was used to test differences between individual schools and by redlining map status. Preliminary data were collected during cold months. No significant difference was observed ($p = 0.178$) between the stressors around schools in redlined versus non-redlined neighborhoods. However, one of the two schools located in a redlined neighborhood did have a significantly greater ($p = 0.0295$)

* Corresponding Author's E-mail: kstewart3661@gmail.com
† Corresponding Author's E-mail: stacy.pettigrew@acphs.edu

In: Neighborhoods: Impact on Child Health and Development
Editors: I Leslie Rubin and Joav Merrick
ISBN: 979-8-89530-834-9

number of stressors compared to the other schools. Statistically significant differences in stressors by redlined status were not observed in this limited analysis. However, a difference in the presence of stressors found between the two redlined schools could be due to differences in the built environment surrounding each school, such as street traffic and green space. Data collection will be repeated in May and September to increase sample size and capture the stressors during warmer months.

Introduction

During the Great Depression starting in 1929, families struggled in their financial day-to-day life due to the decreasing Gross Domestic Product (GDP) and increasing unemployment rates. As a result, approximately 40% of homeowners fell behind on their mortgages (1). In response, President Franklin D Roosevelt (1882-1945) and Congress created the Home Owners' Loan Corporation (HOLC) as part of the New Deal to reduce foreclosures on homes (2). Congress passed the Home Owners' Loan Act of 1933, which allowed the HOLC to provide individuals with low-interest emergency loans over fifteen years to remortgage their homes (2). This opportunity provided individuals and families a way to reduce debts and create a better financial situation in the midst of the larger national financial struggle (2).

'Residential security maps' were created by HOLC to evaluate loan eligibility and were used by banks and other lending agencies in the late 1930s (1, 3-5). While they were designed to aid low-income individuals, the new HOLC maps used economic and racial profiling to determine lending risks in neighborhoods across over 200 cities in the country (1). In addition to housing conditions, accessibility to transportation and parks, and other environmental conditions, residents' race and ethnicity, were used to determine each neighborhood's grade (1). These financial, physical, demographic racial factors were used to grade every neighborhood as A, B, C, or D and color-coded, based on the likelihood that the loans would be repaid (1, 3-5). Areas graded A were considered "best", B graded areas were "still desirable", C graded neighborhoods were "declining", and D graded neighborhoods deemed "hazardous" (5). Areas with a high population of Black, Jewish, immigrant, and/or low-income residents were given a lower grade, and those neighborhoods were color-coded and outlined in red, hence the term 'redlining' (1, 3-5). This redlining practice, endorsed as a federal program, affected generations of residents over the years. HOLC maps were used by banks to determine whether individuals would qualify to receive mortgage and business loans (5). The use of HOLC maps were eventually terminated in the 1960s, however, their use at the time drastically reduced and, in effect, deprived individuals and communities in redlined neighborhoods' the opportunity for economic development at the time, and for the future. The resulting structural discrimination caused long-term effects on communities, including negative health effects (5). Other legacies of structural discrimination and racism are often combined with historic redlining, which serve to magnify negative impact on the affected communities and neighborhoods.

Negative health effects associated with living in previously redlined communities include an increase in diabetes and diabetes-related deaths, heart disease-related mortalities, stroke, asthma, and hypertension among adults (6-8). Additional health disparities include an increased likelihood of preterm birth, a higher prevalence of emergency room related gunshot wounds, and an overall decrease in life expectancy compared to residents of non-redlined neighborhoods (6-8). Neighborhoods that were previously redlined often have other environmental disparities such as less greenspace, increased air pollution, and increased occurrence of extreme heat events, all of which also adversely impact health (6-8).

These health disparities are exacerbated by numerous other social and demographic factors characterized as social determinants of health (7), which often create replicating cycles with intergenerational impact. Limited access to healthy foods, lower educational achievement, and increased poverty rates have been documented in formerly redlined neighborhoods (5, 8-12). Individuals from previously redlined neighborhoods have a lower income compared to individuals who grew up in non-redlined communities, both at the wage and salary level and at the adjusted gross income (AGI) level (3).

Poverty and health are interconnected. Not only are persons living in poverty more likely to have an adverse health outcome, but when these individuals are ill and are forced to take time off from work, they may lose desperately needed income, which can exacerbate their financial insecurity with lasting impact on income for many families in previously redlined neighborhoods (12, 13). This can raise stress levels, which can further compromise health and create a cycle that can be difficult to break.

Stress and academic performance

The Adverse Childhood Experiences (ACEs) study was first published in 1998 and evaluated the effects on children of stressors such as alcoholism and/or drug use by parents, the direct experience of physical and emotional abuse, watching a family member undergo abuse, or having a family member go to jail (14). The ACEs Study observed that increases in childhood stressors at home led to an increase morbidity and mortality in adulthood. In addition, the study found that children who experienced an increase in stressors were also more likely to indulge in risky behaviors as adults (14).

Since the publication of the ACEs Study, numerous studies examining childhood stress and its long-term effects have documented the relationship between childhood stress and many adverse long-term health effects (15-18). Poverty has also been included as an additional measure of stress. One study observed that economic distress and adversity during childhood was associated with an increase of risky behaviors in women (16). Another analysis observed that children living in poverty and just above the poverty level had decreased test scores in school compared to children well above the poverty level (17). These stressful realities could make it more difficult for children to break the cycle of poverty.

In addition to childhood stress, neighborhood stress is also disproportionately present in low-income communities (19). Individuals living in neighborhoods with more stress were more likely to self-report fair or poor health, show distress on the General Health Questions, and have more physical impairments. This suggests that neighborhood stress can disproportionately affect the health and well-being of low-income individuals negatively.

Another type of stress to consider is traumatic stress, which results from a major traumatic event in one's life (20) and leads to an increased amount of day-to-day stress with symptoms described as "reexperiencing, avoidance, arousal, internalizing behaviors, and externalizing behaviors". Traumatic stress can present a significant additional burden on top of the other types of stress previously mentioned.

Children from low socioeconomic communities are also more likely to experience traumatic stress than those from high socioeconomic communities (20). Children who experience traumatic stress perform worse academically during their elementary school years (20). Thus, students from economically disadvantaged neighborhoods are disproportionately affected by stress as a result of adverse environmental factors that they are powerless to change, and which have long term negative effects on their academic performance and professional careers, and ultimately on their potential for future security and success.

Neighborhood violence, which occurs at a higher prevalence in low-income neighborhoods, is also a type of stress that can affect student behavior and academic performance (21-22). Neighborhoods that have a higher incidence of violence tend to have lower standardized testing results in both reading and mathematics (21). Neighborhood violence can lead students to stay home from school out of fear, which may contribute negatively to their academic performance (22).

Local geography

Albany, New York is the capital of New York State (23). It is located along the Hudson River 150 miles North of New York City (23). Albany has a population of approximately 100,000 residents (23). As of 2021, the median household income of Albany was $52,583, compared to New York state's median household income of $74,314 (24, 25). In 2021, 21.7% percent of Albany's population was living in poverty, compared to New York state's level of poverty of 13.9% (24, 25). Albany was one of the many cities across the country where redlining occurred, and resulted in the inhomogeneous distribution of race, ethnicity, income, and poverty throughout the city, which is illustrated by the demographics of public schools in Albany (see table 1).

Table 1. Demographics of Albany, New York and chosen schools, 2022

	Albany	**Giffen Memorial Elementary School**	**Arbor Hill Elementary School**	**Pine Hill Elementary School**	**New Scotland Elementary School**
White	54%	8%	4%	21%	42%
Black	27.7%	54%	67%	43%	26%
American Indian and Alaskan Native	0.1%	1%	0%	0%	0%
Asian	7.5%	8%	3%	7%	10%
Multiracial	7.4%	7%	7%	9%	8%
Hispanic or Latino	9.9%	22%	19%	20%	14%
Median Household Income	$52,583				
Poverty Rate	21.7%				
Economically Disadvantaged		86%	81%	67%	44%

Schools in previously redlined areas

Giffen Memorial Elementary School is located in the South End of Albany, a previously redlined neighborhood. The South End has a lower median household income than the city of Albany and a higher poverty rate. The median household income for the South End is $45,659, with a poverty rate of 25.5% (25). Giffen Memorial Elementary School has almost double the percentage of Black individuals and nearly seven times less White individuals compared to the City of Albany population (Table 1). The higher percentage of Black students and the lower percentage of White students is not unique to Giffen Memorial Elementary School. Similar trends can be seen at Arbor Hill Elementary School, located in another previously redlined neighborhood in the city. The community has voiced concerns about the environmental conditions around Giffen Memorial Elementary School; in particular what students were witnessing on their trip to and from school (26). This research was based on the exploration of those concerns.

Arbor Hill Elementary School is located in the Arbor Hill neighborhood, a previously redlined community, which has a median household income of $22,670 and a poverty rate of 44.9% (27). Similar to the South End, the Arbor Hill neighborhood has a lower median household income and an increased poverty rate compared to the city of Albany as a whole. Arbor Hill Elementary has nearly three times the percentage of Black students compared to the proportion in the overall population of Albany and 13.5 times less White students, similar to the trends at Giffen Memorial Elementary School.

Schools in previously non-redlined areas

Pine Hill Elementary School is located in the Pine Hills neighborhood, located in an historically non-redlined community. The Pine Hills neighborhood has a median household income higher than the median household income in Albany, $70,001, and a poverty rate lower than the average of the city of Albany, 13.2% (28). The percentage of White students is higher than both of the previously redlined schools, and the percentage of Black students is less than two times the percentage of Black individuals in Albany (see table 1).

Similar trends can be seen at the second non-redlined school in the study, New Scotland Elementary School, located in an historically non-redlined community, the neighborhood has a median household income of $66,624 and a poverty rate of 15.7% (29). Both of the non-redlined neighborhoods have a higher median household income and lower poverty rate than Albany and the two historically redlined communities. New Scotland Elementary has the highest percentage of White students than all four schools and the lowest percentage of Black students, both of which are similar to the average found in Albany (see table 1).

Another similarity between the two previously redlined schools, Giffen Memorial Elementary School and Arbor Hill Elementary School, is that they both have a high percentage of students who are economically disadvantaged, which the New York State Department of Education defines as: "Economically disadvantaged students are those who participate in, or whose family participates in, economic assistance programs, such as the free or reduced-price lunch programs, Social Security Insurance (SSI), food stamps, foster care, refugee assistance (cash or medical assistance), Earned Income Tax Credit (EITC), Home Energy Assistance Program (HEAP), Safety Net Assistance (SNA), Bureau of Indian Affairs (BIA) or family assistance: Temporary Assistance for Needy Families (TANF). If one student in a family is identified as low income, all students from that household (economic unit) may be identified as low income." (30). The two non-redlined schools have a lower percentage of students who are economically disadvantaged, as described by the New York State Department of Education (see table 1).

There are discrepancies in the racial composition and economic status within the four schools when compared to each other and when compared to Albany as a whole. The Childhood Opportunity Index, which is supported by diversitydatakids.org and Brandeis University, determines the differences in opportunity that children across the United States have growing up in different cities measured by three broad categories: education, health and environment, and social and economic characteristics (31). In 2020, the Childhood Opportunity Index found Albany, New York had the eighth highest median score for overall childhood opportunity. However, Albany had one of the worst scores out of the 100 worst metropolitan areas for Black children living in low-income neighborhoods. Sixty-nine percent of Black children were living in low-opportunity neighborhoods in Albany. To compound that, Albany was ranked in the top five metropolitan areas to have the worst gap in childhood opportunity between White and Black children. Children with a higher opportunity index are likely to live longer, illustrating a drastic disparity between White and Black children living in Albany.

Based upon those discrepancies and voiced community concern surrounding environmental conditions of some schools in Albany, we aimed to measure whether historic redlining status had any effect on the number of stressors that students experienced on their way to and from school every day. This project aimed to evaluate the difference in stressors that students were witnessing surrounding their elementary school based on whether the school was in a previously redlined neighborhood.

Our study

Four public schools in the Albany School District were selected to be a part of the study. New Scotland Elementary and Pine Hills Elementary are located in previously non-redlined communities, and Arbor Hill Elementary and Giffen Memorial Elementary are located in previously redlined communities (see figure 1).

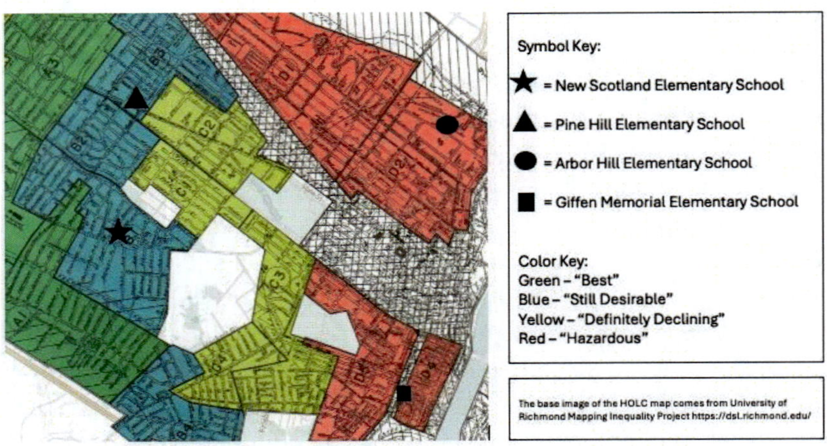

Figure 1. 1938 HOLC map of Albany, New York.

Observational data collection

Observational data was collected. Observational stressors were collected five times for each school on random days for thirty minutes before or after school to determine what students were coming into direct contact with on a regular basis on their way to and from school. Potential stressors included loitering individuals, visible intoxicated or impaired individuals, sleeping individuals, fighting individuals (verbal or physical), a presence of drug paraphernalia, the presence of alcohol, and the presence of tobacco (see table 2).

Table 2. Observed stressor qualification

Stressor	**Visual Qualifications**	**Time Qualifications**
Loitering Individuals	an individual remained in one area without dropping off or leaving with a child	15+ minutes
Visibly intoxicated or impaired individuals	an individual was stumbling *OR* yelling slurred words	5+ minutes
Sleeping Individual	an individual stayed sitting or lying in a position in one area with their eyes shut	10+ minutes
Fighting Individuals	any physical contact between two individuals *OR* if any individuals raised their voiced that caused others to look towards the individuals	N/A
Drug Paraphernalia	any needles *OR* suspicious substances were seen or smelled	N/A
Presence of Alcohol	any alcohol containers or bottles were seen on the ground	N/A
Presence of Tobacco	any packaging on the ground *OR* if individuals were standing smoking *OR* if individuals were stopped at a light or the side of the road visibly smoking	N/A

Observational stressors were determined based on whether the stressor could be seen from the areas where students were being dropped off or picked up. Stressors visible from the observation area were recorded in RedCap version 13.5.1 (2024, Vanderbilt University, Nashville, TN, USA).

Stationary stressor identification

Stationary stressors were identified within a 1000-foot radius of each school using ArcGIS version 10.8.2 (2023, Environmental Systems Research Institute (ESRI), Redlands, CA, USA) to determine what stressors students encountered on a daily basis during their travels to and from school. Stationary stressors were defined as buildings currently used in a way that might cause a stress response to people passing by, including homeless shelters, halfway houses and addiction centers, convenience stores that advertise alcohol and/or tobacco, marijuana dispensaries, and liquor stores.

Data analysis

Types of stressors at each elementary school were reported using descriptive statistics. The differences in presence of stressors by previously redlined and non-redlined status was analyzed using the Kruskal-Wallis test by ranks in RStudio version 12.0 (2023, RStudio Team). The differences in the presence of stressors by school were also analyzed using the Kruskal-Wallis test by ranks.

Our findings

Nine stressor events were observed in person at Giffen Memorial Elementary School. One stressor event was seen at each of the other three schools (see figure 2). The stressors most likely seen were loitering individuals and the presence of tobacco products. A total of ten stressor events were observed at redlined schools compared to two stressor events at non-redlined schools (see table 3). Sleeping individuals, visibly intoxicated individuals, and the presence of alcohol products were not observed at any of the four schools.

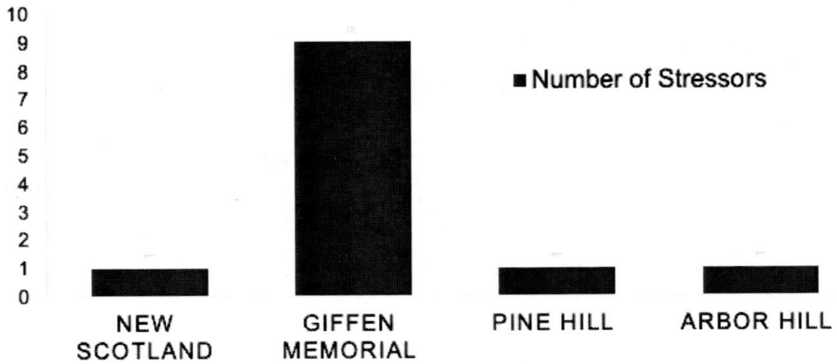

Figure 2. Observed stressors by elementary school, Albany, New York, Nov. 2022 – Dec. 2022.

No stationary stressors were identified around New Scotland Elementary School, two stationary stressors were identified around Pine Hills Elementary School, five stationary stressors were identified around Giffen Memorial Elementary School, and no stationary stressors were identified around Arbor Hill Elementary School (see figure 3). A total of two stationary stressors were identified around non-redlined schools compared to five stationary stressors identified around previously redlined schools (see table 4). Liquor stores and dispensaries were not identified in the immediate vicinity of any of the four elementary schools.

Table 3. Observed stressors by school

Types of Stressors	Non-Redlined		Redlined	
	New Scotland	Pine Hill	Arbor Hill	Giffen Memorial
Loitering Individauls	0	0	1	4
Fighting Individuals	0	0	0	1
Presence of Drug Paraphalia	1	0	0	0
Prescence of Tobacco	0	1	0	4
Total	1	1	1	9
Total Redlined v Non-Redlined	**2**		**10**	

* The following potential stressors were not included in the analysis as they were not observed at any of the four schools: sleeping individuals, intoxicated individuals, or the presence of alcohol.

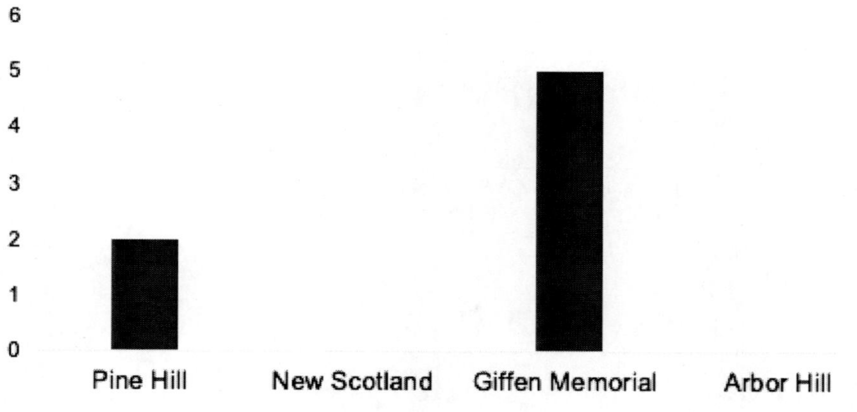

Figure 3. Stationary stressors by elementary school.

Table 4. Stationary stressors observed by school

Types of Stressors	Non-Redlined		Redlined	
	New Scotland	Pine Hill	Arbor Hill	Giffen Memorial
Convenience Stores	0	1	0	0
Halfway Houses / Addiction Centers	0	1	0	2
Homeless Shelters	0	0	0	3
Totals	0	2	0	5
Total Redlined v Non-Redlined	**2**		**5**	

* The following potential stressors were not included in the analysis as they were not observed at any of the four schools: liquor stores and dispensaries.

No difference was observed in the total number of stressors between the two non-redlined versus the two redlined schools (p-value = 0.178) (see figure 4), however a difference was observed in the total number of stressors by elementary school in the redlined areas (p-value = 0.0295) (see figure 5).

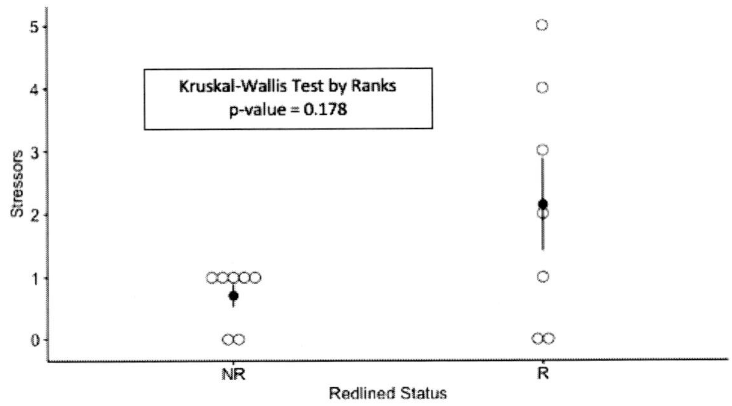

Figure 4. Incidence of stressors by redlined status

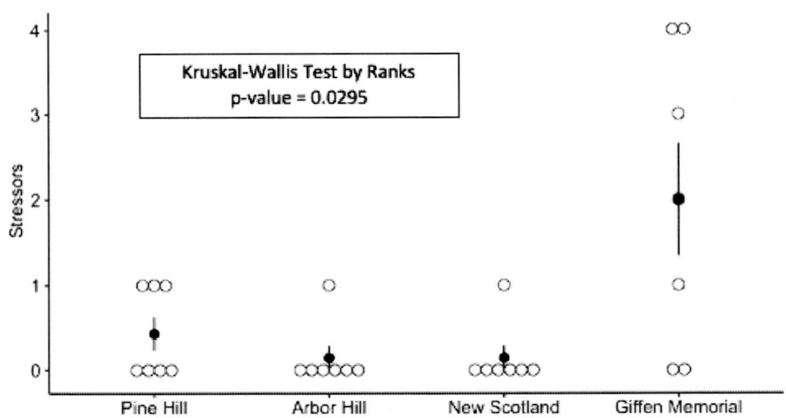

Figure 5. Incidence of stressors by elementary school.

Discussion

It was hypothesized that students who attended elementary schools in previously redlined communities would be more likely to experience an increased number of stressors on their way to and from school. While the results did not show any statistical difference in the number of stressors between the two previously redlined and two non-redlined schools selected for this study, a significantly elevated number of stressors were observed at Giffen Memorial Elementary School compared to the other three schools in the study. Giffen Memorial Elementary School and Arbor Hill Elementary School are both located in previously redlined neighborhoods, yet significantly different stressors were observed. This could be due to aspects of surrounding neighborhoods that were not evaluated in this study. Arbor Hill Elementary School has a larger surrounding green space and is set off from a busy road. The city even built a sidewalk above the busy road that is located close to the school. In addition, Arbor Hill Elementary School is set in a primarily residential area. In contrast, Giffen Memorial Elementary School is located at a busy intersection, with busy roads on three sides of the school and the children are forced to cross the road at the many busy intersections surrounding the school. In addition, there is a limited amount of greenspace surrounding the Giffen Memorial Elementary School.

In other cities on the East Coast, greenspace has been found to be important in children's educational performances. Children who attend schools with an increase in tree cover and active greenspaces have better reading and mathematics standardized test scores (32). This could be one of the reasons why Arbor Hill Elementary School, although located in a previously redlined area, does not have an increase in stressors compared to Giffen Memorial Elementary School.

In addition to differences in greenspace and traffic, Giffen Memorial Elementary is in receivership. In 2015, a law, Education Law – 211-f, was created giving New York State a way to recognize low academic preforming schools in hopes of trying to incentivize the schools to improve their performance on their own (33). Receivership is a status given to schools that perform within the bottom five percent of all public schools on New York standardized tests for three consecutive years (34-36). After being put into receivership, the school is given two years to make "demonstratable improvements" (34). If demonstratable improvements are not made after two years, a school can be taken over by an "independent receiver" who can either make significant changes to the school in hopes of improving performance or shut the school down if they feel that there are no solutions to improve the school's academic performance (33-34). The list of schools placed in receivership is updated every three years, and the latest evaluation was done during the 2021-22 school year (33-34). At this point, thirty-eight schools in

New York State were deemed to be in receivership (36). Two of those schools are in the Albany City Public School District, including Giffen Memorial Elementary School. There is a likelihood that the receivership status of the school could be a result of the significant amount of stress that students of Giffen Memorial Elementary School may be experiencing not only on the way to and from school, but also at home, in the community, and in the classroom, which, cumulatively, could be contributing to the students' and the school's poor academic performance.

Previous research has observed environmental differences between redlined and non-redlined areas (9), and negative health outcomes associated with experiencing adverse childhood experiences and other chronic childhood stress (14, 37). It has also been documented that individuals can experience a stress response within their own neighborhood, in particular with the visual appearance of the neighborhood (19, 38). However, we did not find previous research evaluating the difference in environmental stressors seen around elementary schools based on redlining status using Google Scholar and PubMed searching for the terms: redlining and neighborhood blight, redlining and stress, and redlining and elementary schools.

This analysis examined an aspect of a life that may add another layer of stress to a child's experiences, compounding other stresses they may be experiencing on a daily basis, including family situations. One study observed that with an increase in number of childhood adversities, individuals are more likely to experience multiple adverse physical, medical, and psychosocial experiences as adults (14, 39). Research has shown that for women, cumulative stress, with an ACEs score of 2 or more, is associated with an increase in the rate of hospitalization with autoimmune disorders (40). These findings suggest that cumulative stress during childhood has a long-term lasting impact on psychological and physical health well into adulthood.

This study attempted to fill a gap in previous research by examining how redlining status can contribute to the stressors that children experience on their way to and from school on a daily basis. Analysis of the data revealed that children can experience an increase in stressors around some schools that may negatively affect their school performance. Removing the stressors, particularly the stationary stressors, surrounding elementary schools can lower the stress that children are experiencing and improve their school performance and wellbeing. Overall, this would help reduce the health disparities between children living in historically redlined compared to those living in non-redlined neighborhoods and break the cycle of children's environmental health disparities and promote health equity for all children (see figure 6).

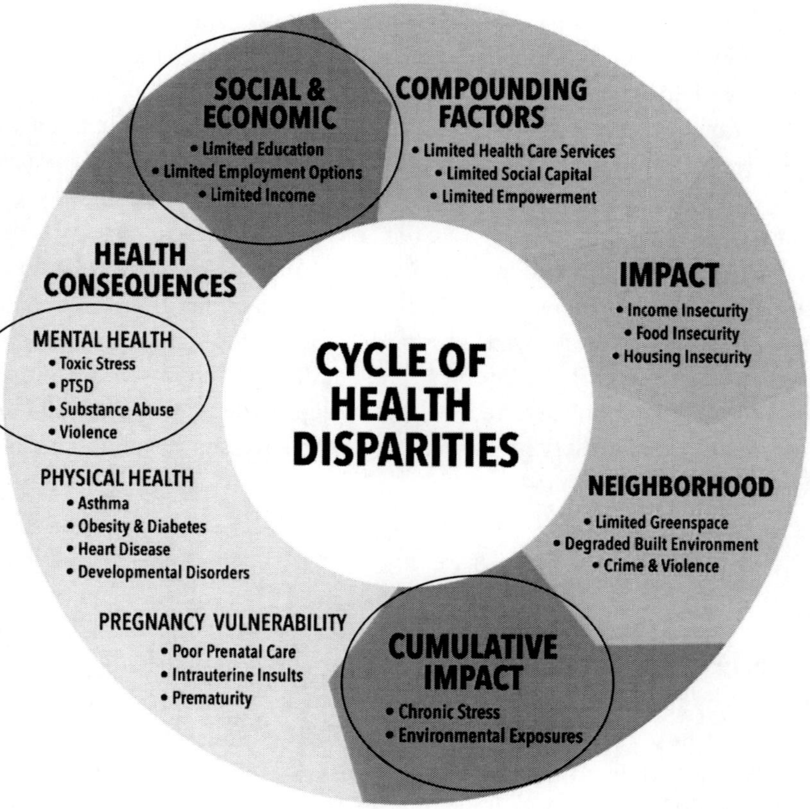

Figure 6. Break the cycle diagram.

More research is needed to evaluate differences in childhood experiences and opportunities and determine what steps can be taken to reduce stress among children as a strategy to reduce children's health disparities and create a change to children's environmental health equity.

Strengths and limitations of the study

The consistency in data collection is a strength, as only one researcher collected data at all four schools. The time of the year that the data were collected could be a limitation, potentially influencing results to the null, because observational data was collected in November and December of 2022, when Albany typically experiences cold, wet weather, with temperatures often below freezing and people are less likely to be outside during this time. Another limitation was the small sample size. A larger sample size in the future may yield statistically significant results.

Additional analyses will seek to compensate for these limitations with data collection during warmer weather. We anticipate that warmer weather will reveal a greater number of observed stressors. In addition, two new schools will be added into the sample, one of which will be found in a previously redlined area and the other will not. One of the added schools will be in receivership, which will allow a better understanding of the number and type of stressors that exist around schools in receivership status, and how those factors may interact with each other. The addition of schools and additional round of data collection in warmer weather will provide a better understanding of the relationship observed between existing stressors around schools in historical redlined communities.

Conclusion

This study sought to break the cycle of children's environmental health disparities by focusing on the built environment surrounding local elementary schools and how that may affect children's stress and health based on the neighborhoods where they grow up, live, learn and play (see figure 6). Reducing childhood stress will result in a reduction of adverse physical and mental health conditions that adults suffer due to the stress that they experienced as children (see figure 6). This study identified additional environmental stressors surrounding an elementary school in a previously redlined neighborhood, and thereby raising awareness of inequity in a school's surroundings that adversely affect children's health, development and education thereby contributing to children's health disparities. It is important that we work towards 'breaking the cycle' to make a positive difference in children's lives by improving the environment and assuring more positive childhood experiences.

Acknowledgements

This project and paper have received editorial support and feedback from the Break the Cycle of Children's Environmental Health Disparities based at the

PEHSU at Emory University and Break the Cycle of Health Disparities, Inc, a non-profit, both in Atlanta, Georgia, United States.

References

[1] Fishback PV, LaVoice J, Shertzer A, Walsh R. The Holc maps: How race and poverty influenced real estate professionals' evaluation of lending risk in the 1930s. NBER Working Paper No 28146, November 2020, Revised October 2021 JEL No J15,N9,R28.

[2] Hillier AE. Residential security maps and neighborhood appraisals: The Home Owners' Loan Corporation and the case of Philadelphia. Soc Sci History 2005;29(2):207–33.

[3] Lynch EE, Malcoe LH, Laurent SE, Richardson J, Mitchell BC, Meier HCS. The legacy of structural racism: Associations between historic redlining, current mortgage lending, and health. SSM-Populat Health 2021;14:100793.

[4] Nardone A, Chiang J, Corburn J. Historic redlining and urban health today in US cities. Environ Justice 2020;13(4):109–19.

[5] Swope CB, Hernández D, Cushing LJ. The relationship of historical redlining with present-day neighborhood environmental and health outcomes: A scoping review and conceptual model. J Urban Health 2022;99(6):959-83.

[6] Egede LE, Walker RJ, Campbell JA, Linde S, Hawks LC, Burgess KM. Modern day consequences of historic redlining: Finding a path forward. J Gen Intern Med 2023;38(6):1534-7.

[7] Jadow BM, Hu L, Zou J, Labovitz D, Ibeh C, Ovbiagele B, et al. Historical redlining, social determinants of health, and stroke prevalence in communities in New York City. JAMA Network Open 2023;6(4):e235875.

[8] Huang SJ, Sehgal NJ. Association of historic redlining and present-day health in Baltimore. PLoS One 2022;17(1):e0261028.

[9] Hwa Jung K, Pitkowsky Z, Argenio K, Quinn JW, Bruzzese JM, Miller RL, et al. Effects of the historical practice of residential redlining in the United States on recent temporal trends of air pollution near New York City schools. Environ Int 2022;169:107551.

[10] Schinasi LH, Kanungo C, Christman Z, Barber S, Tabb L, Headen I. Associations between historical redlining and present-day heat vulnerability housing and land cover characteristics in Philadelphia, PA. J Urban Health 2022;99(1):134-45.

[11] Shaker Y, Grineski SE, Collins TW, Flores AB. Redlining, racism and food access in US urban cores. Agric Human Values 2023;40(1):101-12.

[12] Aaronson D, Hartley D, Mazumder B, Stinson M. The long-run effects of the 1930s redlining maps on children, 2022. URL: https://www2.census.gov/ces/wp/2022/CES-WP-22-56.pdf.

[13] Khullar D, Chokshi D. Health, income, and poverty: Where we are and what could help. Health Affairs 2018 Oct 4. URL: https://www.healthaffairs.org/do/10.1377/hpb20180817.901935/.

[14] Felitti VJ, Anda RF, Nordenberg D, Williamson DF, Spitz AM, Edwards V, et al. Relationship of childhood abuse and household dysfunction to many of the leading causes of death in adults: The adverse childhood experiences (ACE) study. Am J Prev Med 1998;14(4):245-58.
[15] Schmidt KL, Merrill SM, Gill R, Miller GE, Gadermann AM, Kobor MS. Society to cell: How child poverty gets "under the Skin" to influence child development and lifelong health. Dev Rev 2021;61:100983. doi: 10.1016/j.dr.2021.100983.
[16] Braveman P, Heck K, Egerter S, Rinki C, Marchi K, Curtis M. Economic hardship in childhood: A neglected issue in ACE studies? Matern Child Health J 2018;22(3):308-17.
[17] Hair NL, Hanson JL, Wolfe BL, Pollak SD. Association of child poverty, brain development, and academic achievement. *JAMA Pediatr* 2015;169(9):822–9.
[18] Evans GW, Schamberg MA. Childhood poverty, chronic stress, and adult working memory. Proc Natl Acad Sci USA 2009;106(16):6545-9.
[19] Schulz AJ, Mentz G, Lachance L, Johnson J, Gaines C, Israel BA. Associations between socioeconomic status and allostatic load: Effects of neighborhood poverty and tests of mediating pathways. Am J Public Health 2012;102(9):1706-14.
[20] Goodman RD, Miller MD, West-Olatunji CA. Traumatic stress, socioeconomic status, and academic achievement among primary school students. Psychol Trauma Theory Res Pract Policy 2012 May;4(3):252-9.
[21] Milam AJ, Furr-Holden CDM, Leaf PJ. Perceived school and neighborhood safety, neighborhood violence and academic achievement in urban school children. Urban Rev 2010;42:458–67.
[22] Bowen NK, Bowen GL. Effects of crime and violence in neighborhoods and schools on the school behavior and performance of adolescents. J Adolesc Res 1999;14(3):319-42.
[23] About Albany, New York. URL: https://www.albanyny.gov/510/About-Albany.
[24] US Census Bureau. QuickFacts: Albany city, New York. URL: https://www.census.gov/quickfacts/albanycitynewyork.
[25] Explore Census Data. URL: https://data.census.gov/profile/ZCTA5_12202?g=860XX00US12202.
[26] Colon S. "Had enough": Legislator, parents express safety concerns about city mission. Times Union 2024 Feb 11. URL: https://www.timesunion.com/news/article/Had-enough-South-End-legislator-and-16773966.php.
[27] Explore Census. URL: https://data.census.gov/profile/ZCTA5_12203?g=860XX00US12203.
[28] United States. Explore Census Data. URL: https://data.census.gov/profile/ZCTA5_12207?g=860XX00US12207.
[29] Explore Census Data. URL: https://data.census.gov/profile/ZCTA5_12208?g=860XX00US12208.
[30] Enrollment Glossary. NYSED Data Site. URL: https://data.nysed.gov/glossary.php?report=enrollment#:~:text=Economically%20disadvantaged%20students%20are%20those.
[31] Acevedo-Garcia D, Noelke C, Mcardle N, Sofer N, Huntington N, Hardy E, et al. The geography of child opportunity: Why neighborhoods matter for equity. First

findings from the Child Opportunity Index 2.0. URL: https://www.diversitydatakids.org/sites/default/files/file/ddk_the-geography-of-child-opportunity_2020v2_0.pdf.

[32] Kweon BS, Ellis CD, Lee J, Jacobs K. The link between school environments and student academic performance. Urban Forestry Urban Greening 2017;23:35–43.

[33] Fact Sheet 19-8: School receivership. URL: https://www.nysut.org/resources/all-listing/research/fact-sheets/fact-sheet-school-receivership.

[34] Receivership-NYSUT. Future forward. URL: https://futureforwardny.org/stories/receivership#:~:text=Under%20state%20law%2C%20schools%20enter.

[35] New York Consolidated Laws, Education Law - EDN § 211-f. Takeover and restructuring failing schools. URL: https://codes.findlaw.com/ny/education-law/edn-sect-211-f.html.

[36] Receivership. New York State Education Department. URL: https://www.nysed.gov/accountability/school-receivership-demonstrable-improvement-indicators.

[37] Mersky JP, Janczewski CE, Nitkowski JC. Poor mental health among low-income women in the US: The roles of adverse childhood and adult experiences. Soc Sci Med 2018;206:14-21.

[38] South EC, Kondo MC, Cheney RA, Branas CC. Neighborhood blight, stress, and health: A walking trial of urban greening and ambulatory heart rate. Am J Public Health 2015;105(5):909-13.

[39] Dube SR, Fairweather D, Pearson WS, Felitti VJ, Anda RF, Croft JB. Cumulative childhood stress and autoimmune diseases in adults. Psychosom Med 2009;71(2):243-50.

[40] Bürgin D, Boonmann C, Schmeck K, Schmid M, Tripp P, Nishimi K, et al. Compounding stress: Childhood adversity as a risk factor for adulthood trauma exposure in the health and retirement study. J Trauma Stress 2021;34(1):124-36.

Chapter 8

Increased maternal education weakens the link between maternal health during pregnancy and adverse child health outcomes later in life

Margaret Pinder, BSPH[1]
Kyle R Roell, PhD[1,2]
T Michael O'Shea, MD, MPH [3]
and Rebecca C Fry, MS, PhD[1,2,4,*]

[1]Department of Environmental Health Sciences
[2]The Institute for Environmental Health Solutions, Gillings School of Global Public Health, University of North Carolina at Chapel Hill, Chapel Hill, North Carolina, United States of America
[3]Department of Pediatrics, Division of Neonatal-Perinatal Medicine, University of North Carolina, Chapel Hill, North Carolina, United States of America
[4]Curriculum in Toxicology and Environmental Medicine, School of Medicine, University of North Carolina, Chapel Hill, North Carolina, United States of America

Research from the extremely low gestational age newborn (ELGAN) study of children born earlier than 28 weeks' gestation indicates that maternal health conditions during pregnancy are associated with worse health in the offspring. Using extant data from the ELGAN Study we evaluated whether increased years of maternal education between birth and age 15 years moderated the relationship between maternal health conditions and child health at age 15 years. At the time of birth, data were collected about maternal health conditions, including pre-pregnancy diabetes, obesity, hypertension, and asthma. When the ELGAN

---

* Corresponding Author's E-mail: rfry@unc.edu

In: Neighborhoods: Impact on Child Health and Development
Editors: I Leslie Rubin and Joav Merrick
ISBN: 979-8-89530-834-9

participants were born, and when they were two, ten, and fifteen years old, data were collected about the number of years of formal education completed by the mother. Based on data about child health outcomes at 15 years of age, a positive child health index (PCHI) was developed, with higher PCHI indicating more positive health. Among study participants (n = 694), 21% were born at 23-24 weeks of gestation, 46% at 25-26 weeks, and 33% at 27 weeks. Fifty-one percent of participants were male. Sixty-three percent of mothers had reached at least some college education at the time of the ELGAN participant's birth, and 42% had additional years of formal education during their child's first 15 years of life. Three maternal health conditions at birth (asthma, obesity, and diabetes) were associated with worse child health at age 15; maternal hypertension was not associated with child health at age 15 years. In stratified analysis, associations between maternal asthma, obesity, and diabetes and worse child health were weaker among study participants whose mothers completed additional formal education between the child's birth and the child's study visit at 15 years.

Introduction

Extremely low gestational age newborns (ELGANs) are born prior to 28 weeks' gestation are at higher risk for adverse health outcomes at birth and throughout the rest of their lives. At birth, ELGANs are at increased risk for adverse health outcomes including cerebral white matter damage, neonatal chronic lung disease, necrotizing enterocolitis, and other consequences of systemic inflammation. During childhood, ELGANs are at higher risk for neurological disorders such as cognitive impairment, autism, cerebral palsy, and epilepsy (1).

Recently, investigators have focused on factors at birth associated with more positive child health in later life. For studies of positive health, the ELGAN Study investigators developed a Positive Child Health Index (PCHI), an ordinal outcome that accounts for 11 adverse health outcomes: asthma, visual impairment, hearing impairment, gross motor function impairment, epilepsy, attention deficit/hyperactivity disorder, anxiety, depression, cognitive impairment, autism, and obesity. For example, a child with none of those outcomes has a PCHI of 100, while a child with one out of 11 has a PCHI of 90.9, and so on. At the age 10 years the PCHI was used to evaluate the relationship between positive child health and quality of life among ELGANs, as well as predictors of higher or lower PCHI scores (1). As an example, lower pre-pregnancy socioeconomic status and chronic maternal health conditions (pre-pregnancy asthma, obesity, diabetes) were associated with lower PCHI at age 10 indicating poorer health (1).

In this chapter we sought to extend the study of the PCHI among ELGAN participants using the data from the age 15 year follow-up to evaluate how maternal health is associated with positive child health at age 15 years and whether socioeconomic factors could moderate that relationship.

Our study

The ELGAN study is an observational study of the risk of structural and functional neurologic disorders in extremely preterm infants. During the years 2002-2004, women delivering before 28 weeks' gestation in 11 cities in five states in the United States (US) were invited to enroll in the study. A total of 1,506 infants, born to 1,249 mothers, were enrolled and 1,198 survived to age 10 years (79.5%). Among survivors, 1,102 (91.9%) participated in a 2-year assessment, and 889 (74.2%) were evaluated at ten years (2). At age 15 years, we attempted to enroll all surviving members of the ELGAN cohort (n = 1,198). A total of 700 adolescents (58% of surviving cohort members) were evaluated at age 15 years. All procedures for this study were approved by the institutional review boards of all participating institutions.

Maternal and newborn characteristics

Maternal age, education, marital status, eligibility for government-provided medical care insurance (e.g., Medicaid), and racial and ethnic identity were self-reported around the time of birth and again when the child was evaluated at 15 years of age.

The gestational age estimates were based on a hierarchy of the quality of available information. Most desirable were estimates based on the dates of embryo retrieval or intrauterine insemination or fetal ultrasound before the 14th week (62%). When these were not available, reliance was placed sequentially on a fetal ultrasound at 14 or more weeks (29%), last menstrual period (LMP) without fetal ultrasound (7%), and gestational age recorded in the log of the neonatal intensive care unit (1%). The birth weight Z-score is the number of standard deviations the infant's birth weight is above or below the median weight of infants at the same gestational age in a standard data set.

Chronic lung disease (CLD) was defined as receipt of support with mechanical ventilation at 36 weeks post-menstrual age. Cerebral white matter damage, or white matter injury, was defined as the presence of either periventricular echolucency or moderate-to-severe ventriculomegaly determined from newborn cranial ultrasound scans.

Positive child health measures

Participating families completed study visits during which developmental and medical outcomes were assessed. As previously described, at age 10 years (3), clinicians assessed 11 outcomes: cognitive function (School-Age Differential Ability Scales-II Verbal and Nonverbal Reasoning scales) (4, 5); blindness (uncorrectable functional blindness in both eyes) (6); hearing (use of hearing aid, cochlear implant, or special services for hearing impaired person) (6); gross motor function impairment (Gross Motor Function Classification System level ≥ 2) (4, 7); epilepsy (structured interview reviewed by two epileptologists) (8); autism (Social Communication Questionnaire Autism Diagnostic Interview–Revised, Autism Diagnostic Observation Schedule, v.2) (9-11); attention-deficit/hyperactivity disorder, anxiety and depression (Child Symptom Inventory, Parent and Teacher Checklist, 4th ed) (12-14); asthma (medical provider's diagnosis); and obesity (BMI > 95th percentile based on CDC growth charts).

Similar to procedures used to assign the PCHI at age 10 years, information about 11 chronic health outcomes was used to assign a PCHI at age 15 years. The PCHI score of 100% was assigned to ELGANs who had none of the 11 adverse outcomes measured. PCHI score decreased by 9.1% (100/11 = 9.1) for each reported adverse outcome. At age 15 years, the following four child health outcomes were not reassessed because we assumed that if these outcomes were present at earlier ages, they would still be present at age 15 years: blindness, hearing, gross motor function impairment, and autism. To classify study participants as to whether they had epilepsy, we used a validated approach that includes a screening questionnaire completed by a parent or guardian of the child, followed by an epileptologist interview of the parent or guardian whenever the screening questionnaire was positive (8). To ascertain whether the child had asthma, a parent or guardian completed a questionnaire containing the following question: "Since age two years, have you been told by a doctor or other health professional that your child has or has had asthma?". The diagnosis of cognitive impairment at age 15 years was based on the results of assessments using the *Wechsler Abbreviated Scale of Intelligence – II (WASI-II) two-subtest (Vocabulary and Matrix Reasoning) form, which yields estimates of verbal IQ (VIQ), nonverbal IQ (NVIQ) and full scale IQ (FSIQ) (15), and the iPad version of the National Institutes of Health Toolbox Cognition Battery (NTCB)(16.17) to generate estimates of more specific cognitive abilities (e.g., executive function, processing speed).*

We have previously published details of neurocognitive assessments in the ELGAN cohort at 15 years of age (18). For the outcome of cognitive impairment, we included participants who had data on either: (1) Seven of the nine measures of interest, or (2) data on both the WASI-II Verbal and Nonverbal scales, yielding a sample of n = 668). Of these participants, 608 had data on at least seven of the nine measures (593 of these had data on both WASI-II scores), and an additional 60 had data on fewer than seven measures but had data on both WASI scores. Three classes were identified through latent profile analysis. 108 (16.2%) were identified as 'impaired cognition', 352 (52.7%) as 'normal/low normal cognition', and 208 (31.1%) as 'normal/high normal cognition'.

Anxiety, depression and attention deficit hyperactivity disorder (ADHD) were ascertained using the Mini International Neuropsychiatric Interview for Children and Adolescents (MINI-KID 7.0.2) (19), a structured clinical diagnostic interview designed to assess the presence of current DSM-5 and ICD-10 psychiatric disorders in children and adolescents aged 6 to 17 years. We have previously described the results of evaluations of the ELGAN cohort at age 15 years using the MINI-Kid (20).

The diagnosis of obesity was based on measurements of weight and height obtained by study personnel. Body mass index (BMI) was then calculated using the following formula: BMI = Weight (in kilograms)/Height (in meters)^2. BMI Z-scores and percentiles for age and sex were then derived centrally by the study statistician, using the Statistical Analysis Software program based on current CDC growth charts. A BMI centile of 95 or above was considered obese.

Data analysis

We analyzed the relationship between four maternal health outcomes and PCHI, namely hypertension, asthma, diabetes, and obesity. These conditions were chosen because asthma, diabetes, and obesity were associated with poorer children's health at age 10 years (1) and because hypertension is also a chronic maternal health condition associated with the health of offspring. To assess the associations between PCHI and each chosen maternal health outcome, linear regression models were fit. Models were adjusted for sex, gestational age in days, birthweight z-score, public insurance status, and maternal education status. The minimally sufficient set of adjustment variables were defined using a directed acyclic graph.

We further evaluated the associations between PCHI and each maternal health outcome as modified by change between the time that an ELGAN was born and age 15 in the following SES variables: maternal education, maternal marital status, maternal insurance status, and maternal supplemental nutrition and food assistance program (SNAP). To do this, years of education were classified as 1, 2, 3, 4 and 5, corresponding to years of education: less than high school, high school diploma, some college, college degree, and some graduate education, respectively. Maternal education change was defined as any increase between maternal education status at the birth of the infant and the child at age 15 years of age. Change in maternal insurance status from child's birth to age 15 was defined as: higher if insurance status changed from none to public or private, or public to private; lower if insurance status changed from private to either public or none or public to none; and no change if no change occurred. Change in SNAP from child's birth to age 15 years was defined as: higher if SNAP was indicated at birth and no longer at age 15; lower if SNAP was not indicated at birth but indicated at age 15 years; and none if no change occurred. Change in maternal marital status from child's birth to age 15 years was defined as: higher if marital status was unmarried and not living with a partner, divorced, or widowed at birth, and married or living with a partner at age 15; lower if marital status was married or living with a partner at birth, and unmarried and not living with a partner, divorced, or widowed at age 15 years; and none if no change occurred. Upon calculating change variables, multiple linear regressions were run stratified by change status (negative, neutral, or positive, as applicable). Models were adjusted for fetal sex, gestation age, birthweight z-score and each SES variable, excluding the specific one used for stratification in each stratified regression.

Finally, we assessed associations between the individual components of the PCHI outcome, as described previously, and each maternal health outcome, again also stratified by SES change variables. Multiple linear and logistic regressions, where appropriate, were run and adjusted for the following variables: fetal sex, gestational age, birthweight z-score, maternal insurance status, maternal education, maternal marital status, and maternal supplemental nutrition and food assistance program status. All analyses were conducted using R (v4.1.2) (21).

Table 1. Demographic characteristics of ELGAN study participants

Characteristics		**Discharged Alive from NICU (n = 1222) N (%)**	**Age 15 (n = 694) N (%)**
Maternal Age (years)	< 21	174 (14)	80 (12)
	21-35	820 (67)	445 (67)
	> 35	228 (19)	144 (22)
Unmarried Mother		533 (44)	235 (35)
Maternal Education (years)	≤ 12	521 (44)	250 (37)
	> 12 to < 16	276 (24)	153 (23)
	≥ 16	378 (32)	266 (40)
Mother Covered by Medicaid or Another State-supported Medical Insurance		483 (40)	217 (32)
Maternal Race	Asian, Native American, or mixed race	153 (13)	61 (9)
	Black	336 (28)	159 (24)
	White	722 (60)	449 (67)
Hispanic	Yes	147 (12)	57 (8.6)
	No	1068 (88)	609 (91)
Mother's Pre-pregnancy Body Mass Index (kg/m2)	< 18.5	91 (7.8)	47 (7.3)
	18.5 to <30	824 (70)	444 (69)
	≥ 30	256 (22)	154 (24)
Cesarean Delivery		809 (66)	440 (66)
Biological Sex of Infant	Male	638 (52)	341 (51)
	Female	584 (48)	328 (49)
Multiple gestation		365 (32)	236 (38)
Gestational Age (Weeks)	23-24	251 (21)	144 (22)
	25-26	562 (46)	305 (46)
	27	409 (34)	220 (33)
Birth Weight (Grams)	≤ 750	448 (37)	253 (38)
	750-1000	529 (43)	284 (43)
	>1000	245 (20)	132 (20)
Birth Weight Z-score < -2		65 (5.3)	41 (6.1)
Average Daily Weight Gain during neonatal intensive care	Lowest Quartile	301 (25)	156 (23)
	Highest Quartile	308 (25)	167 (25)
Cerebral white matter damage		246 (20)	138 (21)
Chronic Lung Disease		616 (50)	357 (51)

Abbreviations: NICU – neonatal intensive care unit.

Comparison of ELGAN Study participants who were discharged alive from the Neonatal Intensive Care Unit and those evaluated at 15 years of age. Data are number of children (percent of group).

Table 2. Maternal and neonatal characteristics of participants grouped according to maternal health conditions at birth

Characteristics		**Maternal Health Conditions**				
		Asthma	Pre-pregnancy diabetes	Hypertension	Obesity	None of those
		N = 200	N = 43	N = 312	N = 323	N = 829
Birth weight (g)	<=750	83 (41.5%)	23 (53.5%)	186 (59.6%)	152 (47.1%)	336 (40.5%)
	751-1000	86 (43.0%)	15 (34.9%)	97 (31.1%)	126 (39.0%)	323 (39.0%)
	1001-1250	30 (15.0%)	1 (2.33%)	28 (8.97%)	42 (13.0%)	154 (18.6%)
	>1250	1 (0.50%)	4 (9.30%)	1 (0.32%)	3 (0.93%)	16 (1.93%)
Birth weight z-score	< -2	10 (5.00%)	9 (20.9%)	71 (22.8%)	30 (9.29%)	26 (3.14%)
	< -1	33 (16.5%)	8 (18.6%)	90 (28.8%)	50 (15.5%)	82 (9.89%)
	< 0	72 (36.0%)	13 (30.2%)	86 (27.6%)	107 (33.1%)	334 (40.3%)
	>= 0	85 (42.5%)	13 (30.2%)	65 (20.8%)	136 (42.1%)	387 (46.7%)
Gestational age (weeks)	23-24	54 (27.0%)	11 (25.6%)	62 (19.9%)	90 (27.9%)	250 (30.2%)
	25-26	97 (48.5%)	13 (30.2%)	135 (43.3%)	145 (44.9%)	345 (41.6%)
	27	49 (24.5%)	19 (44.2%)	115 (36.9%)	88 (27.2%)	234 (28.2%)
Sex	Female	98 (49.0%)	19 (44.2%)	160 (51.3%)	152 (47.1%)	381 (46.0%)
	Male	102 (51.0%)	24 (55.8%)	152 (48.7%)	171 (52.9%)	448 (54.0%)
Mother's education (years)	<=12	92 (46.0%)	18 (41.9%)	126 (40.4%)	146 (45.2%)	339 (40.9%)
	13-15	60 (30.0%)	13 (30.2%)	88 (28.2%)	106 (32.8%)	138 (16.6%)
	16+	45 (22.5%)	12 (27.9%)	83 (26.6%)	65 (20.1%)	267 (32.2%)
	Missing	3 (1.50%)	0 (0.00%)	15 (4.81%)	6 (1.86%)	85 (10.3%)
Medical insurance from Medicaid	No	104 (52.0%)	26 (60.5%)	177 (56.7%)	174 (53.9%)	468 (56.5%)
	Yes	96 (48.0%)	17 (39.5%)	125 (40.1%)	149 (46.1%)	300 (36.2%)
	Missing	0 (0.00%)	0 (0.00%)	10 (3.21%)	0 (0.00%)	61 (7.36%)
Bronchopulmonary dysplasia, O_2 at 36 weeks	No	73 (36.5%)	12 (27.9%)	99 (31.7%)	116 (35.9%)	354 (42.7%)
	Yes	90 (45.0%)	25 (58.1%)	163 (52.2%)	141 (43.7%)	332 (40.0%)
	Missing	37 (18.5%)	6 (14.0%)	50 (16.0%)	66 (20.4%)	143 (17.2%)
	No	153 (76.5%)	36 (83.7%)	274 (87.8%)	255 (78.9%)	667 (80.5%)

Characteristics		Maternal Health Conditions				
		Asthma	Pre-pregnancy diabetes	Hypertension	Obesity	None of those
		N = 200	N = 43	N = 312	N = 323	N = 829
Cerebral white matter damage	Yes	41 (20.5%)	6 (14.0%)	35 (11.2%)	60 (18.6%)	128 (15.4%)
	Missing	6 (3.00%)	1 (2.33%)	3 (0.96%)	8 (2.48%)	34 (4.10%)
Necrotizing enterocolitis	no/watch/I/II	185 (92.5%)	39 (90.7%)	276 (88.5%)	281 (87.0%)	750 (90.5%)
	Med	0 (0.00%)	0 (0.00%)	4 (1.28%)	3 (0.93%)	11 (1.33%)
	Surg	8 (4.00%)	4 (9.30%)	21 (6.73%)	24 (7.43%)	40 (4.83%)
	Perf	7 (3.50%)	0 (0.00%)	11 (3.53%)	14 (4.33%)	25 (3.02%)
	Missing	0 (0.00%)	0 (0.00%)	0 (0.00%)	1 (0.31%)	3 (0.36%)

Table 3. Change in PCHI at age 15 years of participants with follow-up data at age 15 years grouped according to maternal health conditions at birth and change in maternal education status

Outcomes		Maternal Health Conditions			
		Asthma	Pre-pregnancy diabetes	Hypertension	Obesity
PCHI Score	β (Unstratified)	**-2.836** **95% CI [-5.47, -0.205]**	**-4.661** **95% CI [-9.63, 0.297]**	-0.8337 95% CI [-11.93, 10.27]	**-3.671** **95% CI [-5.60, -1.75]**
	β (NO change in education)	**-4.2891** **95% CI [-7.53, -1.05]**	**-5.633** **95% CI [-11.46, 0.191]**	-1.0787 95% CI [-9.44, 7.28]	**-4.6273** **95% CI [-7.05, -2.20]**
	β (+ change in education)	-0.7735 95% CI [-3.37,1.82]	-3.7127 95% CI [-48.16, 40.73]	-1.4532 95% CI [-3.20, 0.289]	-2.7143 95% CI [-7.90, 2.47]

Analyses were adjusted for sex, gestational age in days, birthweight z-score, public insurance status, and maternal education status when the study participant was born. Bold font indicates statistical significance at $p < 0.05$.

Our findings

The sample size for this study, representing the subjects from the initial study who returned for the 15-year-old follow-up, was 694 (57.8% of participants presumed alive at 15 years of age). Table 1 compares the demographic characteristics of the surviving members of the ELGAN cohort with the demographic characteristics of those who returned for the 15-year evaluation. The percentage of participating children whose mothers had completed high school increased between birth and age 15 years and the percentage of mothers covered by public insurance decreased.

Forty-six percent of children who returned for follow-up were born between 25- and 26-weeks gestational age, and 33% were born at 27 weeks gestational age. Fifty-one percent of follow-up participants were male. Among the entire follow-up cohort at age 15 years, maternal education at the child's birth was at least some college for 63% of participants, and 35% of mothers had single marital status at the time of birth. Three hundred eighty-seven mothers (57.9%) of the subset that returned for the 15-year-follow-up had no change in their education, and the remaining mothers (42.1%) had a positive change in their education over that 15-year period.

Table 2 displays the demographic characteristics of initial ELGAN study participants organized according to adverse maternal health conditions at the birth of an extremely low gestational age newborn. The total n for Table 2 is 1,707, which is greater than the overall n, because mothers with more than one health condition were included in the demographic subgroup for each of their diagnoses. Thus, each column represents all mothers with a diagnosis of a particular health condition, not mothers diagnosed with only that condition.

In simple regressions, adverse maternal health conditions at birth were associated with poorer child health at age 15 (see Table 3). Maternal asthma was associated with an average change in the PCHI of -2.84, indicating a decrement in child health. Maternal diabetes was associated with an average change in the PCHI of -4.66, which maternal obesity was associated with an average change of -3.671. Maternal hypertension was not associated with a statistically significant change in PCHI. We analyzed whether maternal education modified the relationship between chronic illness during pregnancy and child health at 15 years. Three maternal health conditions that had statistically significant associations with poor children's health at age 15 were asthma, obesity, and diabetes. In stratified analysis, the association between maternal asthma and lower PCHI (worse child health) was found only for the stratum with no increase in maternal education between the child's birth and the child's study visit at 15 years; in the stratum with increased education, the association between maternal asthma and lower PCHI was very weak and not statistically significant. A similar moderation of the associations between maternal conditions and PCHI were found in analyses stratified by maternal diabetes and obesity, although the differences between strata with and without increased maternal education were not as large as that found for maternal asthma. There was no evidence that increased maternal education moderated the association between maternal hypertension and lower PCHI.

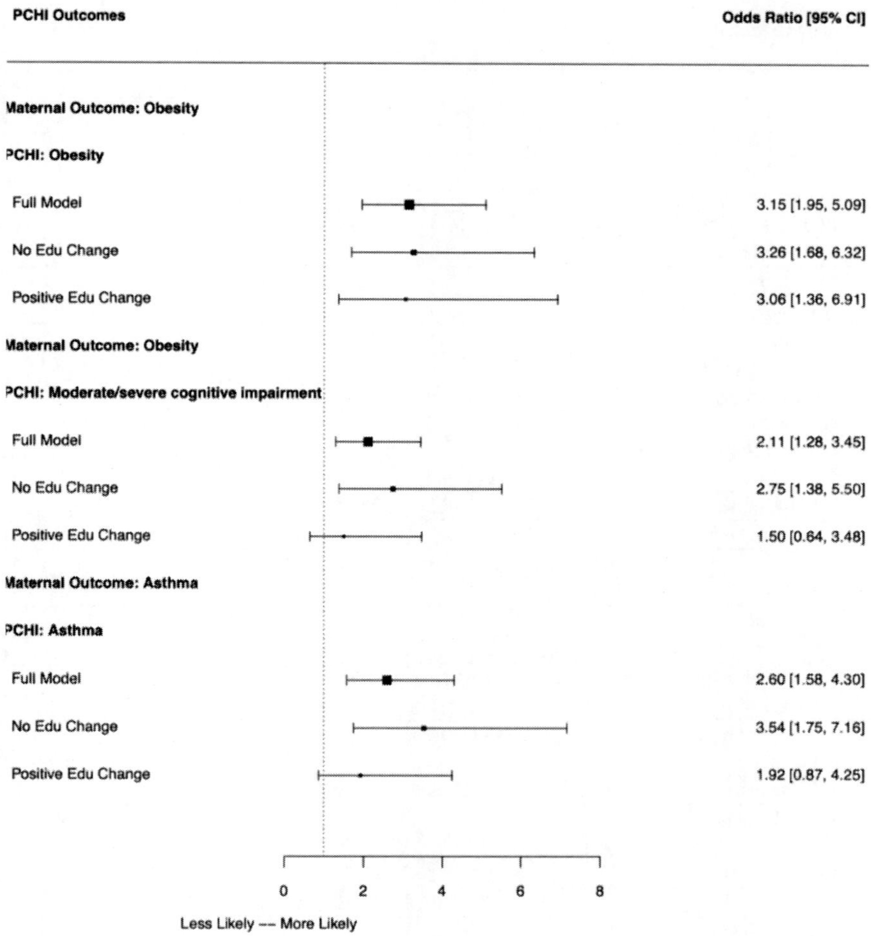

Figure 1. Individual PCHI outcomes and their association with poor maternal health following an increase in maternal education.

Table 5. Antecedents associated with a change in maternal education

	[ALL]	No Change	Positive Change	p.
	N = 597	N=385	N=212	
Maternal Age	29.5 (6.65)	31.4 (6.12)	26.2 (6.27)	<0.001
Maternal Race:				<0.001
White	401 (67.2%)	281 (73.0%)	120 (56.6%)	
Black	138 (23.1%)	71 (18.4%)	67 (31.6%)	
Other	52 (8.71%)	28 (7.27%)	24 (11.3%)	
'Missing'	6 (1.01%)	5 (1.30%)	1 (0.47%)	
Hispanic Ethnicity:				0.088
No	544 (91.1%)	357 (92.7%)	187 (88.2%)	
Yes	53 (8.88%)	28 (7.27%)	25 (11.8%)	
Maternal BMI	25.7 (7.08)	26.1 (7.48)	25.0 (6.27)	0.065
Maternal Education at birth:				<0.001
1 (Less than a high school diploma)	84 (14.1%)	30 (7.79%)	54 (25.5%)	
2 (High school graduate or equivalent)	147 (24.6%)	57 (14.8%)	90 (42.5%)	
3 (Some college)	137 (22.9%)	105 (27.3%)	32 (15.1%)	
4 (College degree)	127 (21.3%)	91 (23.6%)	36 (17.0%)	
5 (Some graduate education)	102 (17.1%)	102 (26.5%)	0 (0.00%)	
Maternal Education at age 15:				<0.001
1 (Less than a high school diploma)	30 (5.03%)	30 (7.79%)	0 (0.00%)	
2 (High school graduate or equivalent)	78 (13.1%)	57 (14.8%)	21 (9.91%)	
3 (Some college)	197 (33.0%)	105 (27.3%)	92 (43.4%)	
4 (College degree)	120 (20.1%)	91 (23.6%)	29 (13.7%)	
5 (Some graduate education)	172 (28.8%)	102 (26.5%)	70 (33.0%)	
Maternal Marital Status at birth:				<0.001
1 (Married)	392 (65.7%)	288 (74.8%)	104 (49.1%)	
2 (Separated or divorced)	22 (3.69%)	9 (2.34%)	13 (6.13%)	
3 (Not ever married but living together)	95 (15.9%)	46 (11.9%)	49 (23.1%)	
4 (Not ever married and not living together)	87 (14.6%)	41 (10.6%)	46 (21.7%)	
5 (Widowed)	1 (0.17%)	1 (0.26%)	0 (0.00%)	
Maternal Insurance Status at birth:				<0.001
no	410 (68.7%)	299 (77.7%)	111 (52.4%)	
yes	187 (31.3%)	86 (22.3%)	101 (47.6%)	
Maternal Nutritional Assistance at birth:				0.078
no	532 (89.1%)	350 (90.9%)	182 (85.8%)	
yes	65 (10.9%)	35 (9.09%)	30 (14.2%)	

To better characterize how increased maternal education weakens the link between maternal health conditions and their child's positive health, the 11 outcomes on which the PCHI is based were considered as separate outcomes. Maternal education weakened the link between maternal health conditions and some PCHI outcomes but did not weaken the link with other PCHI outcomes. For example, maternal asthma is associated with the individual PCHI outcome of asthma in both the full model and when education does not change, resulting in a lower PCHI score (see Figure 1). When there is positive education change, the association between maternal asthma and child asthma was weakened and no longer statistically significant. A similar effect can be seen with the exposure of maternal obesity and the PCHI outcome of moderate to severe cognitive impairment. In both the full model and among mothers without a change in education, maternal obesity was associated with PCHI outcome of moderate to severe cognitive impairment. A change in education has a positive impact on this link. When there is positive education change, the effect is lessened and is no longer statistically significant. Less optimistically, the association between maternal obesity and child obesity was statistically significant and was not modified by a change of maternal education alone; this relationship is also illustrated in Figure 1.

Finally, the project examined other SES modifiers besides maternal education, including change in insurance status between birth and age 15 years, change in maternal marital status between birth and age 15 years, and change in supplemental nutrition and food assistance between birth and age 15 years. None of these SES factors modified the association between maternal health disorders during pregnancy and child well-being at 15 years of age. Compared with change in insurance status, marital status, or receipt of supplemental food assistance, maternal education could be a better indicator or predictor of overall socioeconomic status. In addition, maternal education is distinct in that any change is unidirectional so that only two categories of change are plausible (no change or positive change). In contrast, for the other SES modifiers that we studied, stratifying the cohort resulted in three categories (positive, negative, or no change), providing less statistical precision and power when analyzing effect modification.

Because maternal education significantly improved the PCHI for ELGAN children the study investigated demographic factors that were associated with an increase in maternal education (see Table 5). Mothers who were younger at the birth of the child were more likely to increase their education in the 15 years following their child's birth. Black mothers were more likely to increase their education. Changes in education were most common among women who had no more than a high school degree at the time of birth as compared to all other maternal education categories (some college, college degree, some graduate education). As demonstrated in Table 5, a positive change in maternal education improves a child's PCHI, thereby providing the child with greater likelihood of good health outcomes and improved educational achievement with an increased likelihood of higher income in later life, thus breaking the intergenerational cycle of health disparities for ELGAN children (see Figure 2).

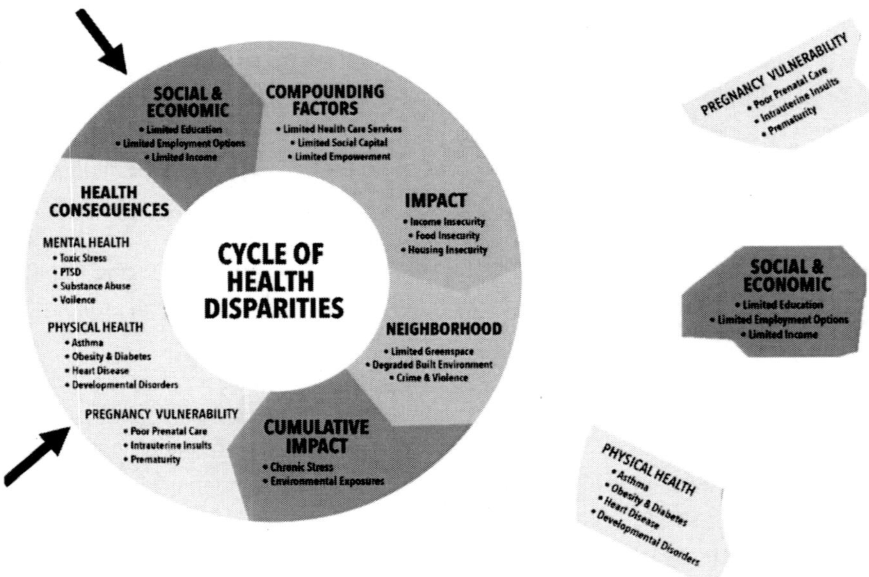

Figure 2. Factors studied in this project that break the cycle.

Discussion

This project identified a pathway for breaking the cycle of children's health disparities by intervening directly where socioeconomic differences link pregnancy vulnerability and offspring health. It is an attempt to weaken that connection with modifiable socioeconomic variables that can be moderated by addressing specific socioeconomic disparities. However, this mechanism for breaking the cycle is limited; for example, the association between maternal obesity and child obesity was statistically significant and was not modified by a change of maternal education alone. The project aims to increase understanding about how social changes during childhood may moderate the relationship between maternal health problems during pregnancy and adverse health outcomes in the child. These results encourage study of the potential interplay between sociological forces affecting reproductive behavior as well as overall health. Preterm birth and associated risks to child health are more common among Black women, as are the chronic illnesses that we studied, emphasizing the disproportionate burden of cycles of disease. We were encouraged by the finding that Black women, women of other historically marginalized racial groups, and women of Hispanic ethnicity were more likely to have an increase in education between birth of an ELGAN and the 15-year follow-ups.

There are many potential mechanisms by which poor maternal health could contribute to worsened child health. Poor maternal health contributes to limited employment options and limited income, and therefore difficulty supporting a child. The impact of these socioeconomic disparities includes food insecurity, healthcare access insecurity, and income insecurity. The results of this study suggest that maternal education addresses this link, perhaps by alleviating the cumulative fatigue and stress of this cycle of health disparities. The specific mechanisms linking maternal education and child health are beyond the scope of this study. However, in a systematic review of mechanisms by which maternal education impacts children's health, major mechanisms cited that have relevance to our study are the following: maternal education could affect health behaviors and thereby improve maternal mental and physical health, overall economic resources and knowledge could increase, and skills and attitudes regarding health could improve (22). Some behaviors, skills, attitudes, and resources that could link grade attainment with infant and child mortality include formal employment, wealth/asset ownership, access to clean water, literacy, knowledge and use of modern contraception, and antenatal/prenatal care (22). Mechanisms such as increased wealth and/or asset ownership could enable a mother with adverse health conditions to employ hired help (e.g., for housekeeping or childcare) or have improved access to healthcare services, resulting in increased mental and physical stamina. Mechanisms such as increased access to antenatal/prenatal care could mediate between pregnancy vulnerability (including premature birth) and environmental, social, economic, and health factors that affect the well-being of pregnant people and infants. These resources could also allow the mother to move to a more advantaged neighborhood where there is less exposure to air pollution, environmental chemicals, and neighborhood violence. It is also important to consider the impact of these lifelong cycles of health disparities for children who live in communities that are disproportionately affected by environmental exposures. Disparities in environmental exposures exist across social determinants of health and these exposures (see Figure 2) influence children's health.

Future directions

In future analyses, we aim to understand the impact of the child's environment more broadly. For example, the current project could be expanded to determine if the established association between maternal health conditions and child health at age 10 and 15 extends to the year 17 data. Potential moderators of the relationship between maternal and child health could be studied in addition to the environmental exposure variables that are currently being collected. These moderators include accentuating factors such as stress, discrimination, and caregiver anger, and attenuating factors like caregiver emotional, informational, or instructional support, as well as the caregiver's overall health. During the ELGAN-ECHO 15-year data collection, the Everyday Discrimination Scale (WEDS) and the PROMIS self-assessment were used to gather self-reported data from study participants regarding many of these potential accentuating factors. There is also the potential to investigate differences in environmental exposures potentially moderating cycles of maternal and children's health that include chemical exposures as well as other potential moderators that can influence children's health, as mentioned above. In future analyses, chemical exposure levels can be included in analyses. The 17-year follow-up data from the ELGAN study includes measures of environmental chemicals, stool and urine sample collection that can be used to assess exposures to environmental toxicants. Other environmental disparities can be studied based on geographic location where study participants reside. Data on ELGAN study participants can be used for analyses that have the potential to increase understanding of the conclusions of the current study.

Strengths and limitations

Strengths of this study are the large and diverse cohort, with longitudinal data collected from birth through 15 years of age. One limitation is the losses between birth (n = 1,506) and follow up at age 15 years (n = 693).

Additionally, analyses were limited to the four SES variables collected at both birth and age 15 years, which do not comprehensively characterize SES. Another limitation is that the results described here might not apply to more recently born cohorts of extremely preterm neonates which include infants born as early as 22 weeks of gestation, a group that is possibly at higher risk for adverse health outcomes than the individuals enrolled in the ELGAN Study.

Conclusion

The results highlight an association between maternal health complications around the time of birth of extremely low gestational age newborns and the children's health outcomes at age 15. We found that an increase in maternal education weakens the link between maternal health complications and children's health. Among the specific PCHI outcomes, moderate-to-severe cognitive impairment and asthma were the child outcomes for which increased maternal education attenuated associations with maternal health disorders during pregnancy.

Acknowledgements

The authors would like to acknowledge the Break the Cycle mentors, especially Dr. Victoria Green. We would also like to acknowledge the ELGAN children and their families who participated in this study, and to the ELGAN Study Investigators. The ELGAN investigators include those from (1) Boston Children's Hospital (Boston MA): Janice Ware, Taryn Coster, Brandi Henson, Rachel Wilson, Kirsten McGhee, Patricia Lee, Aimee Asgarian, Anjali Sadhwani; (2) Tufts Medical Center (Boston MA): Ellen Perrin, Emily Neger, Kathryn Mattern, Jenifer Walkowiak, Susan Barron; (3) University of Massachusetts Medical School (Worcester MA): Jean Frazier, Lauren Venuti, Beth Powers, Ann Foley, Brian Dessureau, Molly Wood, Jill Damon-Minow; (4) Yale University School of Medicine (New Haven, CT): Richard Ehrenkranz, Jennifer Benjamin, Elaine Romano, Kathy Tsatsanis, Katarzyna Chawarska, Sophy Kim, Susan Dieterich, Karen Bearrs; (5) Wake Forest University Baptist Medical Center (Winston-Salem NC): T Michael O'Shea, Nancy Peters, Patricia Brown, Emily Ansusinha, Ellen Waldrep,

Jackie Friedman, Gail Hounshell, Debbie Allred; (6) University Health Systems of Eastern Carolina (Greenville, NC): Stephen C Engelke, Nancy Darden-Saad, Gary Stainback; (7) North Carolina Children's Hospital (Chapel Hill, NC): Diane Warner, Janice Wereszczak, Janice Bernhardt, Joni McKeeman, Echo Meyer; (8) Helen DeVos Children's Hospital (Grand Rapids, MI): Steve Pastyrnak, Wendy Burdo-Hartman, Julie Rathbun, Sarah Nota, Teri Crumb; (9) Sparrow Hospital (Lansing, MI): Madeleine Lenski, Deborah Weiland, Megan Lloyd; (10) University of Chicago Medical Center (Chicago, IL): Scott Hunter, Michael Msall, Rugile Ramoskaite, Suzanne Wiggins, Krissy Washington, Ryan Martin, Barbara Prendergast, Megan Scott; (11) William Beaumont Hospital (Royal Oak, MI): Judith Klarr, Beth Kring, Jennifer DeRidder, Kelly Vogt. This study was supported by the National Institute of Neurological Disorders and Stroke (5U01NS040069; 5U01NS04006), the National Institute of Child Health and Human Development (5P30HD018655), and the NIH ECHO Program (UG3OD023348).

References

[1] Bangma JT, Kwiatkowski E, Psioda M, Santos HPJr, Hooper SR, Douglass L, et al. Early life antecedents of positive child health among 10-year-old children born extremely preterm. Pediatr Res 2019;86(6):758-65.

[2] Helderman JB, O'Shea TM, Kuban KC, Allred EN, Hecht JL, Dammann O, et al. Antenatal antecedents of cognitive impairment at 24 months in extremely low gestational age newborns. Pediatrics 2012;129(3):494-502.

[3] Bangma JT, Kwiatkowski E, Psioda M, Santos HPJr, Hooper SR, Douglass L, et al. Assessing Positive Child Health among Individuals Born Extremely Preterm. J Pediatr 2018;202:44-9.

[4] Kuban KC, Joseph RM, O'Shea TM, Allred EN, Heeren T, Douglass L, et al. Girls and boys born before 28 weeks gestation: Risks of cognitive, behavioral, and neurologic outcomes at age 10 years. J Pediatr 2016;173:69-75.

[5] Beran TN. Elliott CD. Differential ability scales, 2nd ed. San Antonio, TX: Harcourt Assessment. Can J School Psychol 2007;22(1):128-32.

[6] Bright HR, Babata K, Allred EN, Erdei C, Kuban KCK, Joseph RM, et al. Neurocognitive outcomes at 10 years of age in extremely preterm newborns with late-onset bacteremia. J Pediatr 2017;187:43-9.

[7] Palisano R, Rosenbaum P, Walter S, Russell D, Wood E, Galuppi B. Development and reliability of a system to classify gross motor function in children with cerebral palsy. Dev Med Child Neurol 1997;39(4):214-23.

[8] Douglass LM, Heeren TC, Stafstrom CE, DeBassio W, Allred EN, Leviton A, et al. Cumulative incidence of seizures and epilepsy in ten-year-old children born before 28 weeks' gestation. Pediatr Neurol 2017;73:13-9.

[9] Rutter M, Bailey A, Lord C. Social communication questionnaire. Los Angeles, CA: Western Psychological Services, 2003.

[10] Rutter M, Le Couteur A, Lord C. Autism diagnostic interview-revised. Los Angeles, CA: Western Psychological Services, 2003;29(2003):30.

[11] Joseph RM, O'Shea TM, Allred EN, Heeren T, Hirtz D, Paneth N, et al. Prevalence and associated features of autism spectrum disorder in extremely low gestational age newborns at age 10 years. Autism Res 2017;10(2):224-32.

[12] Scott MN, Hunter SJ, Joseph RM, O'Shea TM, Hooper SR, Allred EN, et al. Neurocognitive correlates of attention-deficit hyperactivity disorder symptoms in children born at extremely low gestational age. J Dev Behav Pediatr 2017;38(4):249-59.

[13] Gadow KD, Sprafkin JN. Child symptom inventory 4: Screening and norms manual. Stony Brook, NY: Checkmate Plus Stony Brook, 2002.

[14] Sprafkin J, Gadow KD, Salisbury H, Schneider J, Loney J. Further evidence of reliability and validity of the Child Symptom Inventory-4: Parent checklist in clinically referred boys. J Clin Child Adolesc Psychol 2002;31(4):513-24.

[15] Wechsler D. Wechsler Abbreviated Scale of Intelligence, Second edition (WASI-II). San Antonio, TX. Pearson, 2011.

[16] Weintraub S, Dikmen SS, Heaton RK, Tulsky DS, Zelazo PD, Bauer PJ, et al. Cognition assessment using the NIH Toolbox. Neurology 2013;80(11 Suppl 3):S54-64.

[17] Akshoomoff N, Newman E, Thompson WK, McCabe C, Bloss CS, Chang L, et al. The NIH Toolbox Cognition Battery: Results from a large normative developmental sample (PING). Neuropsychology 2014;28(1):1-10.

[18] Joseph RM, Hooper SR, Heeren T, Santos HPJr, Frazier JA, Venuti L, et al. Maternal social risk, gestational age at delivery, and cognitive outcomes among adolescents born extremely preterm. Paediatr Perinat Epidemiol 2022;36(5):654-64.

[19] Sheehan DV, Sheehan KH, Shytle RD, Janavs J, Bannon Y, Rogers JE, et al. Reliability and validity of the Mini International Neuropsychiatric Interview for Children and Adolescents (MINI-KID). J Clin Psychiatry 2010;71(3):313-26.

[20] Frazier JA, Cochran D, Kim S, Jalnapurkar I, Joseph RM, Hooper SR, et al. Psychiatric outcomes, functioning, and participation in extremely low gestational age newborns at age 15 Years. J Am Acad Child Adolesc Psychiatry 2022;61 (7):892-904.

[21] Team RC. R: A language and environment for statistical computing. Vienna, Austria: R Foundation for Statistical Computing, 2021.

[22] Mensch BS, Chuang EK, Melnikas AJ, Psaki SR. Evidence for causal links between education and maternal and child health: systematic review. Trop Med Int Health 2019;24(5):504-22.

Section two: Acknowledgements

Chapter 9

About the editors

I Leslie Rubin, MD, is originally from South Africa where he trained in pediatrics and emigrated to the United States in 1976. He is currently Associate Professor in the Department of Pediatrics at Morehouse School of Medicine, Adjunct Associate Professor, Department of Pediatrics, Emory University School of Medicine, Director of Break the Cycle Program at the Southeast Pediatric Environmental Health Unit at Emory University (PEHSU), President and Founder of Break the Cycle of Health Disparities Inc, and Medical Director of The Rubin Center for Autism and Developmental Pediatrics in Atlanta, Georgia. He has been involved in the health care of children and adults with intellectual and developmental disabilities since 1977. In 1989, he and Allen Crocker published the first textbook on medical care for children and adults with developmental disabilities with the second edition in 2006. Sadly, Allen Crocker passed away in 2011, but, in partnership with Joav Merrick and others published the 3rd edition: "Health care for people with intellectual and developmental disabilities across the lifespan" with Springer in 2016. He currently directs interdisciplinary clinical programs for children with autism, cerebral palsy and other developmental disabilities and consults to a variety of programs including the Emory University Neurodevelopmental Exposure Clinic (ENEC), an interdisciplinary, research-based program looking at the impact of prenatal exposures on child development and behavior in the context of the social and economic disadvantage and health disparities. Among his awards for various activities, he received the Robert E Cooke Lifetime Achievement Award from the AADMD in 2015 and the Autism Achievement Award in 2016 from the Annual Conference and Exposition of Georgia, and the F Edwards Rushton CATCH Award from the American Academy of Pediatric in 2018, and most recently, was named one of 50 Advocate Heroes over the 50 years of Exceptional Parent Magazine. He is actively involved in the American Academy of Pediatrics as the Chair of the Georgia Chapter Environmental Health Committee and District X CATCH Facilitator for the AAP. He was on the US Environmental Protection Agency Board of Scientific Counsellors focusing on Sustainable Healthy

Communities from 2016-2022 and is now on the National Advisory Council for Children and Disasters. He is also the Chair of the National PEHSU Steering Committee and is on the Advisory Councils of HERCULES, the Human Exposome Research Center at Emory University; and on the National START Advisory Committee, based at the University of New Hampshire. In 2004 he founded the *Break the Cycle* program which addresses children's environmental health disparities by recruiting bright university students to develop creative projects that will *Break the Cycle* and then publish their papers in international journals and books on public health. To date there have been more than 150 students from the USA, Latin America and Africa. The program received the Children's Environmental Health Excellence Award from the EPA in 2016. Email: lrubi01@emory.edu

Joav Merrick, MD, MMedSci, DMSc, born and educated in Denmark is professor of pediatrics, Division of Pediatrics, Hadassah Hebrew University Medical Center, Mt Scopus Campus, Jerusalem, Israel and Kentucky Children's Hospital, University of Kentucky, Lexington, Kentucky United States and professor of public health at the Center for Healthy Development, School of Public Health, Georgia State University, Atlanta, United States, the former medical director of the Health Services, Division for Intellectual and Developmental Disabilities, Ministry of Social Affairs and Social Services, Jerusalem, the founder and director of the National Institute of Child Health and Human Development in Israel. Numerous publications in the field of pediatrics, child health and human development, rehabilitation, intellectual disability, disability, health, welfare, abuse, advocacy, quality of life and prevention. Received the Peter Sabroe Child Award for outstanding work on behalf of Danish Children in 1985 and the International LEGO-Prize ("The Children's Nobel Prize") for an extraordinary contribution towards improvement in child welfare and well-being in 1987. In 2017 appointed a Kentucky Colonel by the Commonwealth of Kentucky, the highest honor the governor can bestow to a person. Email: jmerrick@zahav.net.il

Chapter 10

About the Break the Cycle of Health Disparities Inc

Break the Cycle of Health Disparities Inc. (BCHD) is a private, not-for-profit 501c3, non-governmental organization dedicated to exploring the social, economic and environmental determinants of health in the context of children's health disparities and to use this to promote health equity for all children.

BCHD collaborates with the Southeast PEHSU to produce the annual Break the Cycle of Children's Environmental Health Disparities Program (*Break the Cycle*). *Break the Cycle* is a multidisciplinary academic research and training program that focuses on raising awareness of children's environmental health disparities and cultivating future leaders among university students in the fields of medicine, nursing, public health, law, social work, education and other related disciplines.

Each year, *Break the Cycle* invites students from a diversity of colleges and universities to develop projects that will "break the cycle of children's environmental health disparities". *Break the Cycle* faculty guides and monitors the progress of the students towards compeltion of their projects. The students present their completed projects at a national conference and their work is published in international journals. Over the past 17 years Break the Cycle has engaged over 180 students from over 50 different university departments in 21 states in the USA, as well as students from Latin America, Europe and Africa, that have resulted in the publication of 17 journal supplements. These sets of projects form the basis for this book series.

In 2016, *Break the Cycle* received a Children's Environmental Health Excellence Award from the US Environmental Protection Agency for the achievements of the program.

BCHD has expanded its areas of interest and practice to Break the Cycle of Autism Disparities, Break the Cycle of Climate Change for Vulnerable Children, Break the Cycle of Environmental Degradation, Break the Cycle of Children's Mental Health Disparities, Break the Cycle of Health Disparities among Children from Indigenous Communities, and has launched a Break the Cycle of Health Disparities for Children in Africa program.

Contact

I Leslie Rubin MD

Associate Professor, Department of Pediatrics, Morehouse School of Medicine

Adjuct Associate Profesor, Department of Pediatrics, Emory University School of Medicine

Director, Break the Cycle Program, Southeast Pediatric Environmental Health Specialty Unit, Emory University

President and Founder, Break the Cycle of Health Disparities Inc

Medical Director, The Rubin Center for Autism and Developmental Pediatrics

750 Hammond Drive, Building 1, Suite 100, Atlanta, GA 30328, United States

Email: lrubi01@emory.edu

Website: www.breakthecycleprogram.org

Website: www.therubincenterforautism.org

Chapter 11

About the Pediatric Environmental Health Specialty Units (PEHSU)

The Pediatric Environmental Health Specialty Units (PEHSU's) are an interconnected system of regional centers located throughout the United States that respond to questions from public health professionals, clinicians, policy makers, and the public about environmental health concerns related to children and reproductive age adults. After fifteen years of programmatic operations, collaborations, and a growing desire to protect the health of children and reproductive age adults from environmental hazards, the PEHSU Program has gained the attention and respect of the pediatric and reproductive environmental medical community and families at risk from exposure to environmental contaminants. The PEHSU programs have a critical role in supporting the mission of the Agency for Toxic Substances and Disease Registry (ATSDR) to prevent or mitigate the adverse human health effects and diminished quality of life that result from exposure to hazardous substances in the environment and the mission of the US Environmental Protection Agency (EPA) to protect human health and the environment. The PEHSUs provide a credible, academic, non-commercial source of health information and clinical expertise regarding environmental toxins and their effects on children and reproductive age adults.

ATSDR and EPA established the PEHSUs to increase the capacity of health care providers to identify and treat environmental-related health conditions, prevent exposure to children and reproductive age adults, and communicate health risks from environmental exposures. The PEHSU Network includes teams of medical specialists (pediatricians, medical toxicologists, obstetricians, nurses, nurse practitioners, occupational and environmental health physicians), public health professionals, researchers, psychologists, and educators to provide consultations, trainings, referrals and clinical services to health care providers, governmental agencies and the general public on pediatric and reproductive environmental health. PEHSUs also engage communities and stakeholders in public outreach projects.

The National PEHSU Network helps individuals and communities to make informed decisions regarding environmental health concerns. Common concerns include lead poisoning, fungus or mold, pesticides, phthalates, air quality and school safety. There have also been national responses generated for hazards from wildfires, hurricanes, oil spills, carbon monoxide, mercury spills, de-icer leaks at airports, and industrial pollution.

While Poison Control Centers respond to acute toxic exposures, the PEHSU Network has expertise in long term, chronic low dose exposures, group exposures, and the development and dissemination of public messages. The PEHSU Network partners closely with local, state, and federal agencies and non-profit professional organizations in carrying out this work.

The PEHSUs collaborate with ATSDR and EPA to develop fact sheets targeting clinicians and the public on issues associated with flooding, hurricanes, wildfires, oil spills, formaldehyde, carbon monoxide poisoning, arsenic in foods, medical management of lead exposure, phthalates and bisphenol A, melamine, and other issues. They edit academic textbooks, publish manuscripts, and conduct outreach and educational programs to enhance pediatric and reproductive environmental health literacy.

The PEHSU's provide information online (website: www.pehsu.net) with a variety of materials to educate professionals and the general public in reproductive and children's environmental health through conferences, presentations and social media. PEHSU members serve on national boards and committees to advance collaborative activities and community expertise in environmental health. The PEHSUs train and mentor medical, toxicology, nursing, and other graduate students and provide hands-on opportunities in pediatric environmental medicine and reproductive epidemiology. The PEHSUs have advised first responders, parents, health officials, and school administrators on how to assess and mitigate environmental emergencies and address health-related findings. They have also provided training to establish PEHSUs in Chile, Argentina, Canada, Mexico, Vietnam, and Israel.

The PEHSUs serve to translate research findings into clinical and public health practice. PEHSU faculty are prepared to recognize, treat, and prevent toxic environmental exposures in children and communicate risk, treatment, and prevention strategies in a meaningful and culturally appropriate way.

Southeast PEHSU

The Southeast PEHSU, within the National PEHSU network, serves the southeastern United States and includes Alabama, North Carolina, South Carolina, Florida, Georgia, Kentucky, Mississippi and Tennessee. The Southeast PEHSU is based in the Nell Hodgson Woodruff School of Nursing at Emory University in Atlanta, GA and works closely with Region 4 of the US Environmental Protection Agency (EPA) and the Agency for Toxic Substances and Disease Registry (ATSDR) at the Centers for Disease Control and Prevention (CDC). The team includes Abby Mutic, PhD, MSN, CNM (Assistant Professor and Certified Nurse Midwife), Leslie Rubin, MD (Developmental Pediatrician), Melissa Gittinger, DO (Medical Toxicologist), Rebecca Philipsborn, MD, MPA (Pediatrician), Victoria Green, MD, JD, MBA (Obstetrician Gynecologist), Henry Falk, MD MPH (Formerly Director of ATSDR), Nathan Mutic, MS, MAT, MEd (Educator and Program Administrator), and Wayne Garfinkel, BSCE (formerly of Region 4 EPA). In addition, Benjamin Gitterman, MD (Pediatrician) works with the Southeast PEHSU on the *Break the Cycle* program.

Contact Southeast PEHSU

Abby Mutic, PhD, MSN, CNM
Director, Southeast Pediatric Environmental Health Specialty Unit
Nell Hodgson Woodruff School of Nursing, Emory University
1520 Clifton Road, Atlanta, GA 30322, United States.
Toll free tel: (877) 33 PEHSU or (877) 337-3478
Tel: (404) 727-7980
E-mail: sepehsu@emory.edu
Website: https://www.nursing.emory.edu/pages/southeastern-pediatric-environmental-health-specialty-unit

Chapter 12

About the National Institute of Child Health and Human Development in Israel

The National Institute of Child Health and Human Development (NICHD) in Israel was established in 1998 as a virtual institute under the auspices of the Medical Director, Ministry of Social Affairs and Social Services in order to function as the research arm for the Office of the Medical Director. In 1998 the National Council for Child Health and Pediatrics, Ministry of Health and in 1999 the Director General and Deputy Director General of the Ministry of Health endorsed the establishment of the NICHD.

Mission

The mission of a National Institute for Child Health and Human Development in Israel is to provide an academic focal point for the scholarly interdisciplinary study of child life, health, public health, welfare, disability, rehabilitation, intellectual disability and related aspects of human development. This mission includes research, teaching, clinical work, information and public service activities in the field of child health and human development.

Service and academic activities

Over the years many activities became focused in the south of Israel due to collaboration with various professionals at the Faculty of Health Sciences (FOHS) at the Ben Gurion University of the Negev (BGU). Since 2000 an affiliation with the Zusman Child Development Center at the Pediatric Division of Soroka University Medical Center has resulted in collaboration around the establishment of the Down Syndrome Clinic at that center. In 2002 a full course on "Disability" was established at the Recanati School for Allied

Professions in the Community, FOHS, BGU and in 2005 collaboration was started with the Primary Care Unit of the faculty and disability became part of the master of public health course on “Children and society”. In the academic year 2005-2006 a one semester course on “Aging with disability” was started as part of the master of science program in gerontology in our collaboration with the Center for Multidisciplinary Research in Aging. In 2010 collaborations with the Division of Pediatrics, Hadassah Hebrew University Medical Center, Jerusalem, Israel around the National Down Syndrome Center and teaching students and residents about intellectual and developmental disabilities as part of their training at this campus.

Research activities

The affiliated staff have over the years published work from projects and research activities in this national and international collaboration. In the year 2000 the International Journal of Adolescent Medicine and Health and in 2005 the International Journal on Disability and Human Development of De Gruyter Publishing House (Berlin and New York) were affiliated with the National Institute of Child Health and Human Development. From 2008 also the International Journal of Child Health and Human Development (Nova Science, New York), the International Journal of Child and Adolescent Health (Nova Science) and the Journal of Pain Management (Nova Science) affiliated and from 2009 the International Public Health Journal (Nova Science) and Journal of Alternative Medicine Research (Nova Science). All peer-reviewed international journals.

National collaborations

Nationally the NICHD works in collaboration with the Faculty of Health Sciences, Ben Gurion University of the Negev; Department of Physical Therapy, Sackler School of Medicine, Tel Aviv University; Autism Center, Assaf HaRofeh Medical Center; National Rett and PKU Centers at Chaim Sheba Medical Center, Tel HaShomer; Department of Physiotherapy, Haifa University; Department of Education, Bar Ilan University, Ramat Gan, Faculty of Social Sciences and Health Sciences; College of Judea and Samaria in Ariel and in 2011 affiliation with Center for Pediatric Chronic Diseases and

National Center for Down Syndrome, Department of Pediatrics, Hadassah Hebrew University Medical Center, Mount Scopus Campus, Jerusalem.

International collaborations

Internationally with the Department of Disability and Human Development, College of Applied Health Sciences, University of Illinois at Chicago; Strong Center for Developmental Disabilities, Golisano Children's Hospital at Strong, University of Rochester School of Medicine and Dentistry, New York; Centre on Intellectual Disabilities, University of Albany, New York; Centre for Chronic Disease Prevention and Control, Health Canada, Ottawa; Chandler Medical Center and Children's Hospital, Kentucky Children's Hospital, Section of Adolescent Medicine, University of Kentucky, Lexington; Chronic Disease Prevention and Control Research Center, Baylor College of Medicine, Houston, Texas; Division of Neuroscience, Department of Psychiatry, Columbia University, New York; Institute for the Study of Disadvantage and Disability, Atlanta; Center for Autism and Related Disorders, Department Psychiatry, Children's Hospital Boston, Boston; Department of Pediatric and Adolescent Medicine, Western Michigan University Homer Stryker MD School of Medicine, Kalamazoo, Michigan, United States; Department of Paediatrics, Child Health and Adolescent Medicine, Children's Hospital at Westmead, Westmead, Australia; International Centre for the Study of Occupational and Mental Health, Düsseldorf, Germany; Centre for Advanced Studies in Nursing, Department of General Practice and Primary Care, University of Aberdeen, Aberdeen, United Kingdom; Quality of Life Research Center, Copenhagen, Denmark; Nordic School of Public Health, Gottenburg, Sweden, Scandinavian Institute of Quality of Working Life, Oslo, Norway; The Department of Applied Social Sciences (APSS) of The Hong Kong Polytechnic University Hong Kong.

Targets

Our focus is on research, international collaborations, clinical work, teaching and policy in health, disability and human development and to establish the NICHD as a permanent institute in Israel in order to conduct model research and provide policy aspects in the field of interest.

Contact

Professor Joav Merrick, MD, MMedSci, DMSc

Director, National Institute of Child Health and Human Development, Jerusalem, Israel. E-mail: jmerrick@zahav.net.il

Section three: Index

Index

D

E

F

G

H

I

J

L

M

N

O

P